He's a Porn Addict...Now What?

An Expert and a Former Addict Answer Your Questions

Tony Overbay & Joshua Shea

Table of Contents

Tony Overbay & Joshua Shea

Acknowledgments

Joshua: First and foremost, I must thank my wife, Melissa for her ongoing support. I don't think she realizes just how much my recovery has been expedited by her sticking with me. I would be lost without you, Melissa. Thanks to my kids and the rest of my family for supporting me during those early years of recovery even when nobody was sure of the right thing to say, including me. I'm stronger for having all of you by my side. Much gratitude to Brian Whitney, the best true crime writer in America, for always encouraging me to continue to get my truth out there. There is no Interface greater than friendship. Thanks to the team at MSI Press for believing in this project and being very patient with it. A nod to all of the men and women on WordPress for their stories, answers, and encouragement while writing the book and helping me understand addiction beyond my personal story. Finally, a huge thanks to my co-author and friend Tony Overbay who understood and ran with the concept for this book when I first pitched it. I couldn't imagine a better end result with anyone else, and I'm honored you agreed to this project.

Tony: I am so grateful to my wife Wendy for her continuous support. I am also grateful for my kids, Alexa, McKinley, Sydney, and Jake. They put up with many family home evening meetings where I would begin with the question "So, when's the last time you saw pornography, what was it, and what did you do?" They have no idea how important their love and desire to still spend time with Wendy and me, even as teens, has meant to me. Back to Wendy, she was right there beside me for the ten years I spent in a career that I truly did not feel a passion for, and she was the first one to encourage me to go back to school at the age of 32, with four small children at home. She is truly the coolest person in every room, the rock, the one who can help bring me back to center when my impostor syndrome is screaming. Without her support, I never would have pursued the career change that re-energized me in a way that I never dreamed of. Without her encouragement and support, I never would have started a podcast that now has over two million downloads and has helped more people than I ever could have imagined. Without her support, I wouldn't have created a recovery program that has changed lives. And without those two things, I never would have been in a position to interview Joshua Shea, who has now become a good friend and through the process of writing this book has also played the role of my therapist, helping me deal with deadlines, fear of the unknown, and once again, that darned impostor syndrome. I'm so glad he felt that he could trust me with this project. I believe that his vision of this book was indeed inspired, and it, too, will help countless lives.

Introduction

This book is a unique collaboration between a mental health professional, Tony Overbay, a Licensed Marriage and Family Therapist and Joshua Shea, a former journalist who spent more than two decades struggling with pornography addiction. Usually, the expert sitting in the chair and the person on the couch getting the help don't work together on a project outside of the therapist's office, but we think this is a natural match. (And for those wondering, Josh was never Tony's client—they met on a podcast.)

Tony spends dozens of hours every week working with couples who are at various stages of the therapy process. Many of these couples have struggled with pornography issues. Although you're probably feeling alone in the world right now, you are not. Tony has dealt with women, men and couples who are going through exactly what you are experiencing.

Josh was a pillar of his community when his world came crashing down. A magazine publisher and city councilor, his life changed forever when he was arrested for inappropriate behavior in a computer chat room with a teenage girl in 2013. Trips to inpatient rehabilitation, years of intensive therapy, and a short jail sentence later, he now uses his story to educate others about pornography addiction.

It is our belief that we can provide you with more complete answers to the questions that are festering within you than if you were holding a book by only one of us.

The question probably burning inside of you brighter than any other is the same one we are both asked most often: Is porn addiction real? We answer that question inside the book, but here's an early spoiler: It is 100% real.

Throughout the book, we may refer to an attraction to pornography as an addiction or as an impulse control disorder. The answers often depend on the question, but either way, it is just a label for a condition your partner is dealing with. Practically speaking, it doesn't matter if it's an addiction, an impulse control disorder, or some other label. It is what it is.

Tony works with men every day who try to stop using pornography while their partners look on feeling helpless. Josh knows firsthand it's most likely a behavior that they do not want to continue even if they don't want to talk about it. YOU want to talk about it, and that's why you're reading this book.

There is no miracle phrase, pill, or magic wand. That is the difficulty in quitting the behavior. Chances are that your partner has been lying to his parents, his religious leaders, you, his friends—and himself—for years, which is a big part of the problem.

Some men like the label of addiction because they feel as an "addict" they can then do work that is recommended for addicts, while others don't want to be called addict because it brings up feelings of shame. The great news for both of you is that there are plenty of methods, tools, and programs to overcome the problem. We have seen men's lives changed completely when finally getting this problem behind them. Josh is one such man.

While we hope reading our answers to these oft-asked questions will be incredibly helpful to your journey, we also understand there is no way for us to completely understand all of the backstory of your life as well as your current situation so certain answers may not feel like the correct advice at all times. Our answers will hopefully provide you with a framework to begin processing the multitude of emotions that you're trying to deal with right now. We highly recommend finding a professional, whether it be a licensed therapist, counselor, clinical psychologist, or even a psychiatrist to help you sort through all of the emotions that you're dealing with.

The most foreign, yet strongest emotion you may be feeling is known as "Betrayal Trauma."

There's an old adage that "When the addict gets sick, those around him get sick, too," but pornography addiction is unlike any other addiction. The wife of a gambling addict doesn't wonder what she did wrong in the marriage. The girlfriend of a heroin addict doesn't ask herself if she wasn't enough in the bedroom. That's not the case with pornography addiction.

Betrayal trauma refers to the damage caused when one partner (in this case, your husband or boyfriend) betrays the feelings of safety and trust the other (you) has instilled in them. When the person you rely on for support and survival shows themselves to be not what you expected, it can cut deep. We will delve further into this topic in the book.

In his practice, Tony deals a lot with what is called "gaslighting," and when he was deep into his addiction, Josh felt like he had perfected the art.

If you aren't familiar with the term, it comes from the 1944 movie *Gaslight*. In the movie, the main character turns the gas in his home's lights down slightly each evening and tells his wife that she's imagining that they aren't as bright, eventually causing her to feel like she's going crazy. Gaslighting is a serious issue, but it's also one that can be misunderstood.

When gaslighting is happening, the gaslighter (a husband,[1] in this example) is not only trying to refute what his wife is saying, but he's also trying to make her feel bad for even speaking her truth.

We are grateful that you have entrusted us to help you try and process what is an incredibly difficult time in your life; one that you most likely never anticipated going through. Just please know that there is a lot of help out there, and we're grateful that you've chosen us as part of your discovery/recovery package. The fact that you're seeking help is very important as there are so many people who don't.

Our goal is to provide tools and answers for people who are in relationships where there can be dialogue. If you feel like you are not able to voice your concerns or to be able to express your fears, your hurts, and your pains, then again, we highly recommend that you reach out to a professional.

In Tony's experience, when many women go through the pain of discovery, or disclosure, they are typically met with one of two reactions from their partners. First is the guy who gets it. This is the guy who either got caught in his pornography addiction or pre-emptively confessed to his obsession. Either way, he's the one who says that he will do whatever it takes to make this right with you, with God, with whomever matters to him. He says he'll do counseling, go to recovery meetings, meet with his pastor, let you see his phone, and do whatever it takes because he doesn't want this behavior in his life.

Then there's the other guy. He's the one who says, "Look, you caught me, I'll take care of it, but I don't need you on

---

1   Throughout this book, we refer to the addict as male. This is because almost all of the addicts treated by Tony have been male. In our personal experience, addicts are predominantly male though we know there are many female addicts out there and this information can pertain to their partners as well.

my case every minute of the day, asking me if I'm looking at something or asking to see my phone or my computer." This is the guy who typically is still not fully dealing with the problem. He is prone to gaslighting and unhealthy communication.

As Josh can personally attest, many men ping-pong between the two personality types. Until he spent 17 weeks in inpatient rehab, Josh was much more like the second guy than the first, but he's proof that change can happen. He'll share stories of both sides.

We believe seeing the addict's and the expert's answers side-by-side will give you a unique perspective on the complexities of the problems of addiction and its effects on individual mental health and on relationships.

You are looking for answers, and if you've already reached out to your friends, family, a religious leader, life coach, or a therapist, you've probably received a lot of different answers, and that may leave you even more concerned and confused.

In purchasing this book, you've turned to a former addict and an expert. We truly believe we offer a more complete picture than any other text available. There is nothing like this book on the market, and we are extremely proud of this resource and hope that it will help you in what we know is an incredibly difficult time.

Tony Overbay & Joshua Shea

Chapter 1
My First Questions

How do I know if he's actually an addict?

Tony, the mental health professional

When a client comes into my office to talk about her partner who she thinks is an addict, she'll usually begin to list all the reasons she's sure he's addicted to pornography. Then she'll ask me the question, "How do I really know?"

At this point, I recognize she's doubting herself and questioning her intuition. This usually happens for one of two reasons: either she thinks she's not qualified to make that diagnosis or, most commonly, she doesn't want it to be true. I'll hear the client's entire monologue about her partner's behavior, a behavior that led her to my office in the first place, only to hear her say, "But I'm probably wrong."

What she's really thinking is 'Please tell me I'm wrong.' Chances are, she's not wrong, but there is help, and there is hope.

There are countless definitions of addiction, each with its own little nuances, but for the work I do, I like the definition proposed by the American Society of Addiction Medicine (ASAM.org). It states

"Addiction is characterized by:

• inability to consistently abstain

1

- impairment in behavioral control,

- craving,

- diminished recognition of significant problems with one's behaviors and interpersonal relationships, and

- a dysfunctional emotional response.

Like other chronic diseases, addiction often involves cycles of relapse and remission.

Without treatment or engagement in recovery activities, addiction is progressive and can result in disability or premature death."

But to me, the exact defining of the word *addiction* is largely a matter of semantics. If it's affecting your relationship negatively and you suspect it's an issue that needs to be dealt with, the labeling of "addiction" or "not addiction" becomes irrelevant. If it's negatively affecting your marriage, relationship, or family, it needs to be treated, whatever you want to call it.

I have couples come into my office, and one is adamant that I label the other an addict while the "addict" may be adamant that he (or she) need not be labeled. We can spend the entire session worrying about labels and trying to define addiction, but that's just wasting crucial time that could be spent on repairing their relationship and overcoming the negative behaviors that brought them here to begin with.

This need to label or not label comes up in other areas of my practice as well. In my dealing with clients who may or may not be on the autism spectrum, some come into my office and talk about not being good with social cues, having blind spots, and the like. Finding out they are on the autism spectrum, being labeled autistic is a relief to them because it's finally an answer to explain their behavior. Others walk through the door and clearly exhibit classic signs of autistic behavior, yet repeatedly express that they do not want to be tested or evaluated for fear of being labeled because they're afraid people will treat them differently.

The labeling issue is a universal concern. The label doesn't change who they (you) are, it doesn't change the behaviors exhibited, and it doesn't change what needs to happen next on the path to dealing with the behavior. If your behavior is causing problems in your relationships, whether or not you are clinically identified or labeled as an addict, you need to seek professional help.

Josh, the former pornography addict

The easy answer is that you don't. You've seen the behavior and that should be enough; it does not matter what the label is.

I've been labeled all kinds of things in my life: porn addict, bipolar disorder sufferer, alcoholic, PTSD carrier, narcissistic, depressed, detached, non-empathetic and at some point, they just all started blending together because there are no blood tests for any of them. They are just labels used for diagnostics.

Look at your partner. Let's say he's not an addict. He's still the same person he was five seconds ago. Now, let's say he is an addict. He's the same guy.

There are the typical symptoms you get in all addiction. I'm guessing you're witnessing them in person, but my bigger question to you becomes, "What now changes?"

I'd been told I was an alcoholic for years by many people, and I knew that I was not far from whatever my abstract idea of someone who deals with alcoholism was at the time. I just didn't think I was that far along. I had no idea pornography addiction was a real thing until after I entered recovery.

Was I an alcoholic despite the fact I denied it? Yes.

Was I a porn addict despite the fact I didn't know it? Yes.

Things only changed when I made the decision that it was time for them to change. Yes, there were many factors at work, as I'm sure there is in your life, and I was certainly coerced and shoved into recovery. Looking back, though, I can only thank the people who gave me little choice but to seek help.

You may have a man that wants help, recognizes he needs things to change, and embraces recovery with both arms. You may also have someone in denial, who is either putting up a front in the face of the facts or who genuinely believes nothing is wrong with them. Does it matter if this person is an "addict" according to whatever medical text is in front of you? For the professionals, who have legal, ethical, and diagnostic criteria to follow it does, but for you, it really shouldn't. You know what you're dealing with, regardless of what the insurance company wants to call it.

If the word *addict* scares you, call it a bad habit. Or a compulsion. Or a negative hobby. It really doesn't matter. The biggest question is what you're going to do about it.

Is there a difference between pornography addiction and sex addiction?

Tony, the mental health professional

Similar to the answer to the first question, this one comes back to labels, and whether or not they are relevant. To be clear, until recently, there wasn't anything in either the *American Psychiatric Association's Diagnostic and Statistical Manual of Mental Disorders* (DSM-IV) or the World Health Organization's (WHO) *International Classification of Diseases* (ICD) that talked about sexual addiction or pornography addiction. Recently, the WHO updated the ICD to include Compulsive Sexual Behavior Disorder (CSBD) as a mental health condition. While this designation doesn't exactly meet the standard for addiction, it is definitely the strongest statement made by a body of experts in the field of sexual mental health.

Let me share a very 30,000-foot view of what is happening to the brain when viewing pornography. When a man watches porn, his brain releases the feel-good drug, dopamine. There is some fascinating research around what is called "The Coolidge Effect." The idea is that a male will mate with a receptive female once, and then he can experience a period where he is not interested in mating. However, if you bring in another receptive female, he will then mate again, and so on and so on until he, in essence, can no longer move, almost to the point of death. This phenomenon has been observed in many different species in the animal kingdom.

What is happening is that the "lower brain" or "reactionary brain," was designed to see a female who could possibly help the male bring forth kids to assist in tilling the land and harvesting food. So, his brain pours out dopamine in order for him to hyper-focus on her, do to whatever it takes to convince her that he's her man!

What research now shows is that the lower brain can't differentiate between the real woman in front of it or the pictures and videos it's seeing on a computer screen. So, it will see another "willing female" and pour out dopamine saying, "I need to get her, too!"

But now with an endless supply of "willing females" the brain continues pouring out dopamine basically creating a dopamine binge which kills off many of the dopamine neuroreceptors in the brain. This causes the brain to need to see more or do more to get that same rush as there aren't as many dopamine receptors there to receive the feel-good drug. The addict will start to look for more, sometimes shocking, or twisted, or taboo, things to get the rush. Sometimes, this can lead to people experimenting with people outside of the relationship because they simply want that dopamine rush.

Typically, there is a period of time before a pornography addiction becomes a full-blown sex addiction where the individual will begin to explore what it would take to actually find a partner to have sex with. Sex addicts are not looking for a long-term relationship; they just want a quick fix. I've had many clients in my office explaining the progression from just viewing pornography, to exploring sites that will allow you to connect virtually with someone online, and then to ultimately finding ways to meet up with a real individual for the sole purpose of a sexual encounter.

Whether it's only porn or both porn and sex, the outcome for the individual is the same. It's all about satiating the ever-growing desire and obtaining the requisite dopamine rush that the user needs to feel satisfied. Much like the move from pictures in a magazine to videos or internet pornography, to strip clubs, to massage parlors, to meeting up with an actual partner, the addict is looking for the next rush of dopamine and keeps needing to push the bar higher in order to feel sexually gratified.

With other types of addictions, you often hear the term "gateway." An example would be marijuana as the *gateway* drug to harder substances. While your partner may not be there yet and may never get there, I have seen too many situations where pornography was the *gateway* for acting out sexually. Anecdotally speaking, I have never had a sex addict that hadn't first been addicted to pornography. I have also had clients with severe addictions to pornography that have not acted out sexually.

Josh, the former pornography addict

It's just my preference, but I don't like it when the term "sex addiction" is used to describe my pornography addiction. Let's be honest, when someone says, "That celebrity just admitted to being a sex addict" do you think to yourself that the superstar is dealing with an appetite for pornography or an appetite for intercourse?

I think intercourse, too.

I am not somebody who cheated on his partner, and while I know it will be said elsewhere in this book by both Tony and me, a pornography addiction does not mean that your partner was cheating on you in real life with another person sexually.

I have met plenty of intercourse addicts, and just on the surface, they seem to crave adventure and danger far more than pornography addicts like me, who crave control. I've always been the kind of overly-cautious person who almost never seeks adventure and danger. Sitting in a room looking at pornography in the middle of the night, hoping nobody in the house would wake up was about as daring as I could get.

I'm not here to tell you that looking at pornography, talking to women in chat rooms, or the physical act of intercourse outside of your relationship are all the same on the level. I've met women who consider pornography use to be as bad as cheating. This is one of those gray-area situations you'll have to decide for yourself if you find pornography use escalated.

"Sex addiction" has, by default, become the catch-all term. I find myself telling people that I went to "sex addiction rehab" in Texas in 2015 despite the fact I think only two out of a dozen or so in the program actually had intercourse addictions. If statistics continue to skew in the current direction, there are going to be far more porn addicts than intercourse addicts in the world, and maybe then we'll start to get separate billing. I hope that the World Health Organization's recognition of Sexual Impulse Disorder in mid-2018 will also move us in a direction of no longer lumping sex addicts and porn addicts together.

As a former addict, I see a big difference. I believe my wife does, too.

Was he this way when we first got together?

Tony, the mental health professional:

Typically, spouses ask this question because they want to know one of two things:

1) How did I not see this until now?

2) Did I somehow drive him to this behavior?

The first is a loaded question. If you've been together for many years, there are so many ways you are both different from each other and so many ways in which you have both changed over the years. Is he the same person you fell in love with and married? Probably not 100%. But neither are you. I can tell you based on seeing hundreds of individuals and sitting with them collectively for thousands of hours, that this is not an addiction that pops up overnight. However, it is an addiction that is steeped in guilt, shame, secrecy, and isolation, all of which are developed over time as the addiction progresses.

If this addiction was there prior to when you met and were dating, your partner probably hoped that the sex life you would eventually share would be enough to take away any desire to view pornography or masturbate. Unfortunately, unless addicts begin doing serious recovery work, simply getting into a monogamous relationship is not enough to address the addiction. Acting out sexually, whether in a committed relationship or a one-night stand, does not satisfy the addictive nature of pornography use.

I believe that the addiction has very little to do with the spouse, although I can understand how difficult that may be for the spouse to accept. This addiction began with the husband's early exposure to pornography, to him then becoming "sexualized" young, where the wiring of the brain began to view a lot of his life through a sexually-charged lens. Addiction also springs from a well of unmet needs and lack of connection. He's most likely felt disconnected from his work, his schooling, his health, and his relationships, and his brain is turning to pornography whenever he's not feeling good about himself or his situation. Over time, turning to pornography has become habitual and instinctual.

Sometimes, I share with clients that no one typically picks up smoking in their 20s or 30s, and the concept is similar with pornography. There is early exposure that leads to an addiction of turning to porn for stress relief, to numb out, and to cope with problems. By the time an addict is married, lookoing at pornography is how he reacts to any and all of the above stressors.

Josh, the former pornography addict:

Depending on how long you've been together, your husband either was already there or the pieces were in place, and the tendency just hadn't blossomed into something terrible yet. I maintained my addiction for over 20 years without recognizing it could be classified as such. Once it was brought to my attention, it still took six months and hundreds of hours of therapy before I was willing to truly accept it.

Reading between the lines, you could be asking the question "Is this my fault?" The answer, even if he'd never seen porn before meeting you (which is unlikely in 99.99999% of cases), is that none of this is your fault. This isn't a blame situation for you...or him.

If he's an addict, it means he's sick. He doesn't have to come to terms with it to actually be sick. Just because I came to accept my porn addiction as a mental illness did not mean it began at that moment of revelation. It means I saw it was there with clear understanding for the first time. Denial or acceptance has little to do with the condition.

I've seen statistics that say 90-95% of people with sexually focused addiction issues have some kind of trauma from abuse that took place early in life. It doesn't have to be sexual in nature, but it often is.

I was not in the critical stage of pornography addiction when I first met my wife in 2002. I had long been in the ongoing stage where usage would cyclically spike and wane for at least a decade by that point. I don't think I reached the critical phase when things started to go off the rails until 2013.

Were the pieces all there when I met her? Probably, but like a stew, they needed to be mixed and boiled to the proper temperature. I think we're all capable of a lot of negative things that never quite reach that breaking point.

Looking at it objectively, I can't point a finger at her for any of it. These were my issues. She is to be commended for keeping the family together not just during the first 11 years of my marriage before I entered recovery, but also even today for shepherding her flock through those years when I was at inpatient rehab or doing my jail time. Life is probably as easy for us as it ever has been now, but through it all, none of my addiction issues had anything to do with her.

He probably was that way when you got together. It's just that other influences have let it get out of hand. You didn't cause any of this even if he claims the exact opposite.

Isn't it normal for most guys to like pornography?

Tony, the mental health professional:

The quick answer is yes. Based on the statistics we have, the average guy likes porn. I think, though, it brings up a deeper question, "Is it healthy for guys to like porn?" (Or, is it healthy for guys to watch porn?) I think that answer is no.

In today's society, porn is one of the biggest parts of the formula when it comes to men objectifying women. I understand survival of the fittest, evolution, and the need for there to be attraction toward your mate, but the way that women are objectified in the world's culture goes well beyond anything Darwin was talking about.

In the faith-based world, God instructed Adam and Eve to multiply and replenish the earth. We know that one of the reasons men and women were made to find each other attractive was to encourage reproduction. So when working with men, I like to start by saying that it's normal to find the opposite sex attractive, but there's a line where finding someone attractive quickly crosses over to objectification.

Pornography encourages 100% objectification of the people involved, and I think that that attitude seeps into every facet of the lives of those involved in pornography in any way, and especially of those who feel that they are addicted, or if they won't admit they are addicted, we'll say those who feel that they can't quit viewing pornography for long periods of time.

I have a lot of men come into my office, either for individual therapy or for couple's therapy, and on the surface they have no idea how often they objectify women. It is such a part of their inner thought process that they don't even realize they're doing it. Their brains are in an almost constant state of thinking sexually about women, from what the breasts of a woman on the other side of the room look like to different things they'd like their partner to do in the bedroom.

In terms of pornography addiction, it usually becomes about a sub-genre of pornography objectification. It's not just about looking at breasts and butts. It can go from what's more typically thought about when we think of sex, to objectifying a woman's feet and wondering what they look like in terms of pornographic thoughts. Sure, it's just somebody's feet, but it's still objectification.

Speaking in terms of evolution, let's look at it this way. You're driving down the street and you see somebody attractive. It's not objectification to think "attractive person." What you do with the next thought is more telling. Do you dwell on a certain body part? Do you wonder what they would look like without their clothes? Do you picture them performing sex acts? Or wonder what it would be like to have sex with them?

Our thoughts that come naturally can turn into sexualization and sexualization can quickly turn into objectification. There is a distinct line that is often crossed, and when it is crossed, you begin to feed the beast.

Josh, the former pornography addict:

Well, if the numbers of guys who watch porn are anywhere near accurate—and there's no reason to think they aren't—then yes, it is normal, meaning that more men look at porn than not. But, let's remember that normal is really just a synonym for the word "average."

The average guy also likes football but isn't obsessed. Some men like football to the point that they pay thousands of dollars for NFL season tickets and paint their chest to show their support, even in snowy, 2-degree weather. Then there is a population of men who don't like football at all.

Who is normal in this scenario? The non-obsessed fan is the most "average" of the three according to statistics. Who is next average? The non-fan or the chest painter? It's probably the guy who isn't obsessed.

Move this analogy to drinking. I recently saw a survey from 2015 that said 56 percent of adults drank alcohol in the previous month. That would mean the "average" adult drank alcohol. How many drank it once or twice at dinner or a social function? Probably far more than the number who have a hardcore alcohol problem.

Is it normal to like porn? Statistics would say yes. Is it normal to obsess over porn? No.

This can't really be like other addictions, can it?

Tony, the mental health expert:

Yes and no. The negative effects on an addict's outside life can range from very minimal to life altering, regardless of the addiction. If you're missing work because you're putting a needle in your arm or playing video games, you're still missing work. Your addiction may get you fired, and it doesn't matter what the addiction is in this case.

On a cellular level, drugs and alcohol will obviously cause negative physical effects to your body simply because that kind of addiction is introducing foreign chemicals to the body.

On a dopamine level, it's the same—but different. The dopamine surge that comes with playing a video game is on the same level as somebody who is craving a piece of pizza and gets it, based on the research I've looked at. There's a reward given to the pleasure centers of the brain by satisfying that urge.

The dopamine rush from something like heroin or cocaine is ten times that of the video game, even for the addict. I would guess that pornography is somewhere in the middle.

Now, the problem with addiction is that dopamine hit, whether it was a giant one with heroin or a tiny one with Fortnite on an Xbox, quickly dissipates. Over time, you need to blast those neuroreceptors in the brain with even more of whatever it is that is giving you pleasure, because the amount of dopamine that once gave pleasure doesn't quite cut it anymore.

I don't want anybody reading this to think, "Well, at least he's not addicted to crack or meth," as a way of justifying or minimizing pornography addiction. You probably wouldn't be ten times worse if he was doing that. Conversely, you're not 10 times worse than you would be if he was "only" addicted to video games. Or are you?

This is one of those questions that I urge people not to get too attached to in terms of measuring the true cost of their partner's addiction.

As I'll state throughout this book, repeated viewing of pornography warps one's sexuality. It takes away from an opportunity to truly connect with a spouse, or partner, at a level that so many men believe does not even exist, a level where they are fully present with the person in front of them and not thinking about, or needing, pornographic images in order for them to be intimate with their partner.

Josh, the former pornography addict:

It wasn't until I was well into my second stint at inpatient rehab that I started to believe that not only were my alcoholism and porn addiction actual diseases, but I was not all that different from the people who had addictions to things I had no issues with, like heroin or gambling.

I came to accept the fact I have an addictive personality. There are plenty of reasons and theories as to how I got here, but I don't think the 10-year-old kid who had to finish the Zelda video game faster than any of his friends or who had nearly a quarter-million baseball cards by age 14 was all that different than the guy who found solace in Red Bull & tequila or on a computer screen featuring naked women two decades later.

If there were hardcore drug addicts in my life, I never knew it. When I got to the first rehab center in Palm Springs to deal with my alcoholism, I was met with people who I would have honestly crossed the street to avoid. They were dirty and made bad choices. They didn't have the moral willpower that I did. I knew how to say no to crack and meth.

Being forced into an environment with all of these people, I came to recognize I had more in common with them than the people who I rubbed shoulders with in the "real life" I left behind. These people knew pain, were master manipulators and found a way to soothe the demons that raged inside of them. Their demons were usually similar to mine, even if our coping mechanisms were not.

I used alcohol and pornography interchangeably. Obviously, if I was at a professional social function, I couldn't access pornography on my phone, so I'd drink up. If I was alone at home, the computer was always there to fill a need. Late at night, when my wife and kids were fast asleep, I could engage both of my addictions.

There are obvious differences in the legality of substances, and drugs will do other harmful things to your body, but I truly believe addiction is addiction is addiction. My fight these days is just as much about not falling into another addiction as it is staving off the ones I've identified. Recovery includes learning not to engage with new behaviors and substances.

He says that looking at *Playboy* or going to a strip club with friends isn't porn addiction. Is he right?

Tony, the mental health expert:

Like many of these questions that focus on the label of "addiction," it really comes down to a matter of semantics. How do you feel about the fact that he looks at *Playboy* or goes to look at women dance naked at a strip club? Forget the articles, forget the friends…if a husband said it wasn't addiction to me in a session, I'd tell him it's not about addiction, it's about objectification. His line of thinking is rationalization and justification, be it addiction or not.

How do you feel when he looks at the women in a magazine or when you're sitting at home knowing that he's out looking at a 22-year-old gyrating on stage? If you're sharing your emotional truth that it bothers you with him and he tells you that it shouldn't, he's not having any empathy toward what the situation is like for you. Lack of empathy, not coincidentally, is one of the hallmarks of addiction.

Addict or not, I would label the husband's attitude and behavior as a problem. It's certainly not the way to build a healthy relationship. I see some couples where the word "addiction" is thrown around because she is worried where things are headed. She may not think he's an addict now, but has seen a rise in some kind of behavior giving her concern.

An interesting question to ask yourself would be how you would feel if suddenly the twice-a-week *"occasional"* trips to the strip club with friends became frequent visits to the nearby casino with his buddies to play craps or roulette? What if he told you that wasn't an addiction?

There aren't a lot of easy answers, but your feelings and intuition will generally guide you to be rightly concerned in a given situation.

Josh, the former pornography addict:

He's mostly right, but if he is an addict, his answer is more of a rationalization by comparing himself to non-addicts.

Reading *All About Beer Magazine* and going to a brew pub with friends once in a while isn't going to make him an alcoholic, but if he already is one, it's like throwing gasoline on a fire.

It's impossible to tell exactly what ingredients are going to make one person an addict and the next a recreational user because they are often the same formula. It's like the phenomenon where two people grow up in the same household and one ends up a criminal while the other is a captain of industry. You just can't tell how things are going to end up, although if addiction has been established, it is possible to avoid potentially damaging situations. Don't bring a gambling addict to a casino and don't take a porn addict to a strip club.

Sex Addicts Anonymous has a system of three circles that indicate how severe a behavior is in relation to succumbing to the addiction. The middle circle, which lives between the outer circle of healthy behavior and inner circle of full-blown addiction is often called "the slippery slope."

Middle circle behaviors for me could include being isolated late at night, drinking alcohol or watching sexy movies on HBO or Cinemax. I haven't been in a strip club in over a decade, and they had little-to-no relation to my porn addiction back then. They were social events with friends. They wouldn't register as negative behavior for me because it's just not something on my radar.

If he's the kind of guy who enjoys going to these places solo, getting a lot of lap dances and revving his engine so he can come home to enjoy porn, strip clubs would be in the middle circle for him. It may even be considered inner circle if it really gets out of hand.

Looking at *Playboy* wasn't a middle circle behavior for me in my early days of porn addiction in the 1990s. It was inner circle. It was *THE* problem, along with VHS tapes, until the Internet entered my life. I don't think I've seen a *Playboy* in nearly 20 years, but I still make sure to stay away from them, as it will always be a middle circle behavior.

I feel like with many questions in this book, there is a question-behind-the-question. Are you actually asking, "Is it okay I don't like these things and think they are a problem?" The answer to both of those questions is a resounding, "Yes."

If you don't like his behavior and/or you think that certain things he does contribute to the problem, you need to express this to him. There are many men, even if they are struggling with an addiction, who will respect your wishes when it comes to spending money to watch naked women jiggle in front of them.

You can set boundaries where you don't allow certain magazines in your home, or you can tell him that you don't approve of his behavior. He may be a guy who apologizes and stops engaging in those behaviors or someone who laughs in your face and ignores you. How you deal with that is a different issue we tackle elsewhere.

He always seems to stare at women too long. Should that have been a sign?

Tony, the mental health professional:

We talked a little bit about this earlier. It's not the first look that is the problem. It's the second look that comes in just a blink of an eye afterward.

I find that this question—and many others like it—generally comes immediately after a woman discovers the addiction, and is less about the behavior in addiction and more about asking themselves, "If I noticed this, would we not be in the position we find ourselves right now?"

That's not a productive train of thought. Naturally, you're trying to make sense of how you got here, what, if anything, your role was, and what, if anything, you could have done differently to produce a different result. Asking yourself 1,001 "What If" questions is normal, but it's not productive. You can't change what happened. You are where you are now, and you have to look forward.

Imagine it exactly like putting a jigsaw puzzle together knowing you don't have all of the pieces. Let's say you put what you have together and it's a picture of your partner, and he's holding something, but you can't tell exactly what it is because those pieces are missing.

Those missing pieces may show that he's holding a basket of cookies. They may also show that he is holding a gun. It may only be a small piece of the overall puzzle missing, but it changes the entire story of the puzzle. You can do some real damage to yourself if you're trying to figure out all of the gaps. Dwelling on the past won't change anything, but focusing on the present and looking toward the future can help both you and your partner on the path to recovery.

Josh, the former pornography addict:

I'm sure that you're replaying the movie in your head of all the time you've ever spent with him that you didn't recognize he was an addict. You are wondering what you missed. If you can, stop playing the film. It's like a news clip. It's already happened and there's nothing you can do to go back to change those events.

You can shape future events and have an influence on where your life, both together and as individuals, goes from here. Try your best not to dwell in the past; it's easy to get stuck there.

He probably had dozens of little "tells" that were part of his addict behavior. Odds are he also didn't recognize most of them.

If I'm driving down the street, especially in summer, and a woman is pretty, I'll look at her. I think that's perfectly normal. I have a friend that I met through Sex Addicts Anonymous who tells me that when he was in his addiction, which had more voyeuristic tendencies than mine, he would see the pretty girl, turn the car around to look at her again, then turn around to look at her again, then go through that routine a few more times. Years ago, if a friend did that, I may have laughed and thought that he was putting on a show of being obsessed. Now I recognize it's probably a red flag.

Don't make yourself crazy over-examining every little thing he does and trying to draw a line back to his addiction. Instead, figure out which behaviors make you personally uncomfortable and share them with him. If he's obviously leering, drooling and whistling when a pretty woman walks by, that's not only insulting to you, it's embarrassing for everyone involved.

I had a therapist who once said, "You have three seconds to think anything you want as a function of human nature. Beyond that, you're making a choice."

If he's making the choice to stare down women and you don't like it, say something. The women probably don't like it either.

I've heard the term "gaslighting" used in this situation. What does it mean?

Tony, the mental health professional:

Gaslighting is basically when the betrayed asks a question of the betrayer, and the betrayer is able to take the question and flip it around to either ask a similar (yet often nonsensical) question of the betrayed or provide an answer that leaves the betrayed feeling crazy for even suggesting it or stupid for asking the question in the first place.

It's manipulation, manipulation, manipulation. For example:

Wife: Why were you late coming home last night?

Husband: I went and grabbed a beer with friends.

Wife: Lisa said she saw you coming out of an adult movie theater yesterday after work.

Husband: When did she tell you this?

Wife: Last night before you got home.

Husband: Does Bill know his wife is going to adult movie theaters?

Wife: What? She was on the outside.

Husband: I was with my friends, including Bill. Do you want to call him and check?

Wife: No.

Husband: You should, or are you making that part about Lisa up? Are you lying?

Wife: No. No, I'm not.

Husband: Doesn't it seem strange she'd see me and not her husband? Especially since neither of us were at a movie (strip club, book store, etc.). We got a beer.

Wife: But she said…

Husband: In this world of 8 billion people, do you think she could have made a mistake? Call her and see if she's totally sure. She'll laugh at you.

Wife: Never mind.

Husband: I can't believe you'd think I'd even go to one of those places.

Wife: Sorry.

I would wager that the husband was by himself at a theater and the wife's friend absolutely saw him. He knew if he threw a bunch of rapid-fire questions at her that questioned the reality of the situation that she would back off. You know that she didn't forget about it when the conversation was over. She probably walked away wondering if her husband could have been telling the truth and she was jumping to conclusions by listening to her friend. That's classic gaslighting.

I have people trying to gaslight me in my office every day. It's the go-to defense mechanism for personality disorders like narcissism and addiction. If there's a tendency toward narcissism, this is an especially effective tool in their arsenal. They can gaslight with a single blank stare. When I try to bring them back to the initial question, I'm usually told I'm an idiot, not a good therapist, or some other personal attack.

I could write an entire book about gaslighting, but the thing to walk away with is that you need to be confident in your truths. What if you saw him walking out of the theater instead of your friend? Could he still talk his way out of it? Be confident that you, not he, lives in a world of truth. It's important to understand how gaslighting works and how damaging it can be to your relationship. Be aware when your partner uses this form of manipulation so you don't get caught in its trap.

Josh, the former pornography addict:

I know Tony will handle the technical side of gaslighting, so I'll just handle the been-there, done-that side.

Gaslighting is me making you think that you're crazy for asking me questions about being a porn addict. Gaslighting is me manipulating you into doubting your own good sense of what is happening in front of your eyes.

It's me telling you that I'm getting better and taking care of my problems, so you live on the fumes of false hope. It's about saying what I need to say and doing what I need to do in any given situation so I can continue to be an addict and take the spotlight off of myself.

Gaslighting is the control I have over you. I know you don't want to leave this marriage or relationship. I know you love me. I know you worry about how you'd deal with finances on your own or what would happen to the kids if you took some kind of stand about my condition. I know all of these things and I will use all of them to my advantage.

I want you to stop asking questions and telling me what to do, and I want to be left alone to engage in my unhealthy behavior. I'll do what it takes to make that happen because I'm an addict. Porn, sex, gambling, drugs, alcohol, food—it doesn't matter the addiction. As long as you're standing in the way of me getting what I want, I'll do what I need to do to move you out of the way, even if it's hold you mentally and emotionally hostage. That because I'm an addict.

You may read this and think to yourself, "What an evil person, my man isn't like that," but I've described just about every addict I've ever met.

Tony tells me the term comes from an old movie, but it should be a magic show, because gaslighting is the No. 1 illusion in any addict's box of tricks.

We all learn how to lie and manipulate in life, it's just that the addict, by sheer means of practice and necessity, gets really good at it. Maybe that's why I did well in business and politics. I said what I had to say to get what I wanted.

There were times when I would lie about something and think to myself, "Holy crap. That sounded legit! I could be an actor!"

I look back now and realize it wasn't a compliment.

I know he's looked at gay porn and other strange porn. Does that mean he's gay or have a problem?

Tony, the mental health professional:

No, not necessarily. My first thought goes to the stereotypical setting in a locker room at the gym where there may not be individual shower stalls or people are walking around naked. Are you gay because you take a look? No.

The world of porn is so disturbingly vast that people can find themselves on websites that have links and thumbnails to things he has no immediate interest in seeing, but curiosity takes hold and he finds himself clicking through almost anything. While I don't think it's healthy to look at pornography, I think that curiosity can be expected, especially with an addict.

I've had plenty of addicts in my office who have told me that "normal" pornography no longer does it for them, so they have to go looking for something else. See the earlier description of the Coolidge Effect.

I think you can look at it the same way you might look at eating from a buffet in Las Vegas. If you were just ordering off a traditional menu, you'd probably get something that you knew for sure you would like. But when you have a buffet, you can try a little bit of this and a little bit of that. If you find something you like, you can go back for a little more.

Now, with that said, I have also had clients who were closeted gay men living the life of a straight man. Usually some shame-based activity happened when they were young, or they know that living an open gay life would only ostracize them from friends, family, and church. For a lot of these men, if they weren't already acting out with other men, gay porn was their release.

If he's an addict, I would be more apt to think he's just looking at something to satiate his desire for porn and not be too quick to draw conclusions for what that means in his "real life."

Josh, the former pornography addict:

It may express some kind of latent or oblivious interest, but it also may just be that he is at a place of addiction where the "normal stuff" doesn't do it for him anymore. If you want to laugh, shudder, or have some kind of reaction in between, visit a pornography site and take a look at all of the exotic categories of pornography that exist.

Since it is an addiction, the addict needs to constantly tweak the pleasure sensors in the brain, but with repeated use, the pleasure sensors eventually become numb. Watching a man and a woman have sex becomes watching a man and two women, then maybe five people.

Once watching people have sex isn't enough, they may move onto things like roleplaying, BDSM, and same-sex interactions. He may not be at all interested in pursuing anything he sees on a computer screen in real life. I know that I wasn't.

I got to the place that I needed to see extreme pornography that was well outside the norm of what people generally watch, but I can also say that I never wanted anyone to urinate on me and I was never attracted to someone two-to-three times my age in real life. If there's a genre, I probably watched it at some point, but 98% of it would have scared the hell out of me anywhere but on a computer screen.

I tended to prefer genres that were either real-life scenarios or where the actors were good enough to fool me into thinking it was candid. It made the porn "real" instead of poorly acted films with the same people and horrible music. The idea of somebody getting caught doing something they shouldn't raised the stakes and flicked my pleasure center. I hadn't yet figured out my issues connecting the "danger" of the porn I looked at to the "danger" I felt as a child in sexually-charged situations. It really didn't matter what was on the screen as long as it wasn't an actor in a fake set-up.

Ironically, I didn't like danger in my adult sex life. If I wasn't behind a locked door with my wife in a place that nobody could hear us or walk in on us, I couldn't enjoy sex. The idea that my child may wake up on the other side of the house and hear something put a damper on our experience for a long time. I preferred nights my kids spent at their friends' houses or nights where we happened to be in a hotel, because there was nobody I cared about on the other side of that wall.

You'd never guess I was so careful about who heard me based on what I looked at on my computer. I presented a completely different picture based on my porn viewing profile.

Could he be gay? Sure. There's probably a lot you don't know about his sexual preferences well beyond his favored gender. Just don't use what he's been looking at as a guide to who he really is. As it was with my case, it could be exactly the opposite.

Tony Overbay & Joshua Shea

Chapter 2
Understanding and Coping with Feelings of Betrayal

How did he manage to conceal it all so well and deceive me for such a long time?

Tony, the mental health professional:

You may have just found out, but more than likely there have been years of this pattern of behavior on his part that have led to either his disclosure or your discovery, and during these years there has undoubtedly been a tremendous amount of guilt and shame on his part.

Guilt can be a good emotion, because it can cause someone to evaluate a situation and motivate them to do something different. But when shame kicks in, that's the voice that tells you, "You're a horrible person and you'll never overcome this. People are going to know you're a fraud, or that you're disgusting if they ever find out about this." Pornography is the type of addiction that for most individuals is laced with guilt and shame, evolving into an addiction fueled by isolation because they don't want anyone to know anything about it

In my practice, I can't count the number of times I've had a couple in front of me and the wife (who has no idea about her husband's use) says something like, "My friend

Tina caught her husband Bob looking at pornography. I can't believe guys look at that, it's disgusting! She kicked him out. If that happened to me, I'd do the same thing!"

Even if he wanted to disclose his use at this time, he's hearing a message that his addiction is going to end his marriage. He's going to have to leave. His life as he knows it will be over. All of this leads to even more guilt and shame, which will just lead to more isolation.

For him, concealing has been part of a routine. When I work with clients trying to break pornography addiction, often times we're trying to break that routine, which has been solid and foolproof for years.

Most men have a mental checklist as part of their routine: Make sure she's gone, lock the door, close the blinds, make sure the phone is nearby. There's also a routine for when he is finished, and neither are haphazard. They are methodical about things. They craft a world where they can do this and nobody is going to know. As the addiction grows, they may get more extreme with things like burner phones or installing apps to hide their behavior. The depth of guilt and shame associated with this addiction have caused him to work diligently to keep it hidden from you.

Josh, the former pornography addict:

My wife was under the impression I looked at porn once in a while. She was never a prude and believed an occasional glance at porn was just something guys do. Unfortunately, she had no idea the extent to which I watched, nor the reasons for my use, which put me far into the addict category.

I've been a porn addict since the very first time I saw hardcore pornography at 11. By the point I met my wife, around 15 years later, I knew how to hide my porn use from my parents, girlfriends, roommates, friends and every other human I came into contact with. Hiding my use from my wife was never a challenge, nor did it ever feel like a deceitful behavior because I'd been doing it so long.

When I reached the most critical stage of my porn addiction, I had sunk to such lows (including communicating with women in chat rooms) that even if I had wanted to come clean about my behavior, the potential cost of disclosure seemed too great. I thought she would leave if I told her what was happening.

If you're a typical partner in what you believe is a healthy relationship, your life is not consumed by what your husband or boyfriend is doing when you're not around. Even if you have relationship problems, pornography addiction is not one of those things that's we're programmed to look for in our partners. It's easy to hide what the other person is not looking for.

Have you ever noticed the moon in the sky in the middle of the day? It's almost always there, but you really don't see it unless you're actively looking for it. Were you actively looking for a pornography addiction? I know my wife was not. I had enough other issues on the surface that she needed to deal with. Spending the time and energy to dig deep and look for things that weren't obvious was not something she did.

The revelation that he successfully hid this from you for a long time should not make you feel like you weren't paying enough attention. It should not make you feel stupid or ignorant. It should not make you feel like you were played for a fool. He hid his behavior because he knew you would not approve and that it would hurt you. He likely also felt a great amount of shame using it to meet whatever gap it filled in his mind, body and soul. This doesn't excuse the behavior, but hopefully once you can internalize this, you'll realize the bigger question is why he needed it in the first place.

Some people say I don't want him to disclose everything to me. Are they correct?

Tony, the mental health professional:

"I want to know everything you did" is one of those statements I hear regularly in my therapy sessions with couples.

There is a modality of therapy where the husband and wife start putting out their truths.

It's viewed as an emotional bid to be vulnerable. The idea is that they are sharing their heart with their partner, but it's done knowing that the other person loves and cares about them and wants to know their truth.

So, there's disclosure from the spouse and all of a sudden we're in this world known as betrayal trauma, where the wife is going back and trying to put everything together. This is the point at which I hear phrases like: "My whole marriage has been a sham," or, "I can't trust anything he says or does now."

For the wife, it often becomes, "I want to know more. I want to know everything. I just want answers to these questions."

But then what I see over and over again is that one question leads to another question leads to another question, and then the wife may come back later and say, "OK, hey you said this and that made me think of this, this, and this."

If his story changes at all it can be devastating to the wife because you're already dealing with an individual who feels like they have been betrayed. Even now during the disclosure the husband's story is changing, so in her mind he must still be lying, even if he's not intentionally lying.

At this point, her head starts spinning—I had a client call this the "dryer" because it's like a clothes dryer—the more he tries to disclose, the worse it gets and the more amped up she gets and the more her head is spinning. He sees this and at some point may get frustrated and lash out. All we've done with disclosure is create more damage.

Disclosure can be a tricky ongoing piece of therapy. If I have a male client who has an issue with looking at women's chests, we may work at having him look at women's eyes. During a couple's therapy session his partner may want to know if he still finds himself looking at women's chests. If he answers that he's doing a lot better and really focusing on looking elsewhere (or looking at their eyes), she may still want a definitive answer, yes or no. If he admits that he has slipped once or twice—or several times—typically the partner's reaction is something like, "I can't believe you still do that. How am I ever going to trust you?" This type of reaction, though understandable, leaves him feeling he's in a no-win scenario.

To avoid this, when I sit with a couple, we talk about some rules of engagement.

We agree we all want to know the truth, but we also know the addict, or the betrayer, is probably not going to be able to say these things in a way that will satisfy his partner.

The disclosure needs to take place for healing, but with that said, I would encourage the couple to seek help from a professional who understands how to work with betrayal trauma, or else it's possible you may cause more damage.

Remember, to the addict it may feel good to unload their burden, to confess; it's finally out in the open! But to the spouse, this is most likely new. There's a concept in the world of betrayal trauma called a "staggered disclosure," which means that every time the addict comes to his wife and remembers more, or shares more, she is retraumatized. I would highly recommend seeking help from a qualified professional who is trained in working with betrayal trauma.

Josh, the former pornography addict:

Think about an article on the Internet or in the newspaper. You can generally get the gist of the story by looking at the headline, the first paragraph and a photograph. At that point, you ask yourself if you really need to know the whole story.

I think that if you do not want to hear the details of his pornography usage, you need to let him know up front. He could be the kind of person who wants to unburden himself and come clean. Stop him. He has not earned that right. He can tell a therapist. On the other hand, if you are the kind of person who wants to know every last detail, I urge you stop and strongly consider the ramifications, because you can't unhear a detail you really didn't want to know.

Your husband's pornography addiction is like a piece of steak. You can examine the whole, then cut it into 100 bite-sized pieces for "easier" digestion, but it's still the same steak. Like a steak that has a fatty bit, some of the pieces of his addiction story are going to be harder to stomach than others.

If you want to know everything, I believe you have that right. If the disclosure of his addiction is recent, he's probably still in a state of shame, embarrassment and denial. He will likely rationalize and minimize his behavior when it comes to details, falling back on his skills of deceit and omission to make things seem healthier than they were. That's muscle memory. He's been acting this way for so long, it's what comes natural.

My wife was smart about it. She made the decision to protect herself and only got the headlines. There are total strangers who know certain aspects of my tale that she doesn't because she avoided specifics, whereas when I give interviews on the subject, I go into depth. She also knew that she wanted to attempt to move forward with me and learning lurid details would only cause deeper anger and resentment that she may not have been able to get over.

When my first book came out, she made the choice to not read it despite the fact that I told her there were very few graphic details. She made that decision because that time in our relationship is one she doesn't want to re-live, and I don't blame her for it. It wouldn't surprise me at all if she didn't read this book. That's her right.

You may think you're prepared and that you're the kind of person who "needs to know." Just think twice before asking for it all.

Does he love porn more than me?

Tony, the mental health professional:

At some point in his life, he turned to porn as a coping mechanism. He wasn't feeling connected to his job, his kids, his health, his church, his parents, and his spouse. He turned to porn because he didn't necessarily know how to connect to his life. Most likely he fell into a habit of turning to porn because he didn't have the tools to become a better husband, father, or employee; he didn't have the discipline to get in better shape or write the great American novel. He turned to porn as a coping mechanism.

Not everything has to tie back to childhood, but I've found that when you have early exposure to pornography, somewhere under age 11 or 12 (the average age of first exposure continues to trend down, it now sits somewhere between 8 and 11) you tend to become sexualized. Back before porn was at everyone's fingertips, the term sexualized typically meant some form of molestation, but now we understand that early exposure to porn has similar effects.

I like to put it this way. When exposed to porn early, the young developing brain now sees even Mrs. Johnson, the third-grade teacher, no longer as simply Mrs. Johnson, but as a woman with breasts and curves, and he begins to fantasize about her. His neighbor, who maybe hasn't been exposed to porn early, still innocently sees her as his 3rd grade teacher.

I feel like when you see early exposure in this light, it begins to make clear how developing brains can take off from the same location and begin to head in two completely different directions.

The point is, in most cases, he was sexualized long before he ever met you. He developed an addiction to pornography drawn by his need to cope with a variety of stressors in his life.

It's important to remember that pornography is a symptom of a larger problem and becomes the go-to coping mechanism. Perhaps he is in a career he hates, he doesn't like the shape he's in or he feels like he doesn't know how to be a good husband or father. There are so many things they don't like about themselves, so porn becomes that outlet and that coping mechanism. The brain locks into it because then it doesn't have to deal with the real problems. Pornography is full of stimulating images and ends in an orgasm, so there is a moment of feeling great. There's a complete escape from reality, from the difficult and hard things he's dealing with. It's not about a lack of love.

Josh, the former pornography addict:

No, he doesn't. That's an easy answer. Throughout my entire recovery, be it inpatient rehab, 12-step groups, court-mandated support groups or in my travels meeting people both online and in real life who struggle with porn addiction, I have never found one who loves the pornography more than he loves his partner.

The weird reality is, he probably doesn't like porn at this point, but like an alcoholic with a drink or a gambler with a set of dice, he can't stay away. His mind has convinced him that he needs the porn to function. I'll leave the neuroscience to Tony and other medical professionals, but if you've never had an addiction, it's impossible to understand the unwavering, irresistible pull it has over the mind. When people say that addiction is a choice and not a disease, I tell them to thank their lucky stars they have the luxury of the ignorance to have that opinion.

My attraction to pornography and the reasons I used it were almost the exact same reasons I became an alcoholic. Both helped my anxiety, were soothing, and made me feel in control—all of the typical reasons an addict uses. There was nothing unique about me as an addict, but many non-addicts see someone struggling with addiction as having a failure of moral character, not somebody who is sick and in pain.

I can make a list of 1,000 things I LIKED more than porn. I can make a list of 1,000 things I LOVED more than porn. But I can't make a list of more than three things I thought I NEEDED more than porn when I was in the middle of the illness.

As I've mentioned elsewhere, he probably went to such lengths to hide his addiction from you precisely because he loves you. If he didn't, he wouldn't care what you thought. He wouldn't care about your reaction or bother to think about the pain it would cause. It seems counterintuitive, but that's an addict's thinking for you.

There's a reason (probably several) why he developed the addiction and it has nothing to do with the quantity or quality of his love for you. His mind screams a need for pornography that he can't quiet until he feeds the beast. His need for porn should never be confused as a lack of love for you. It is a completely separate thing. It has nothing to do with you.

Did porn ruin our sex life or did our sex life drive him to porn?

Tony, the mental health professional:

There is no question in my mind that porn warps sexuality and can lead to an unhealthy sex life. There is a phenomenon known as The Coolidge Effect. In a nutshell, it's been discovered that with just about every species of animal, sexual interest decreases with the same partner over time, but males may exhibit renewed interest with new, receptive sexual partners, even if the original partner is still receptive and available.

Think about pornography. It's an unending supply of new females who are always willing to meet his needs. Even though it's not real life, images in a magazine or on a computer screen can prompt The Coolidge Effect. This is because the lower brain can't tell the difference between something that is really in front of you and something that is not actually there but on a screen.

It all has to do with a chemical called dopamine. The best explanation I've seen comes from Dr. Kevin Majeres, a member of the faculty at Harvard Medical School, on his blog, PurityIsPossible.com:

"Dopamine is the drug of desire—when you see something desirable, your brain pours out dopamine, saying "Go for it! Do whatever it takes!" Dopamine fixes your attention on that desirable object, giving you your power of concentration...

So when someone clicks and sees a new pornographic image, his lower brain thinks this is the real thing, this is the lady he must win over with all his might, and so he gets an enormous dopamine flood in his upper brain, causing a wild amount of electrical energy.

This first exposure to a new female who is a potential mate wasn't something that happened a lot to our ancestors; maybe only once in their lives; so the brain thinks this is a big deal. It doesn't know that now the game has completely changed: it doesn't understand that these are virtual females only; so with each new one it causes another flood of dopamine, time after time, click after click, as long as he continues. It's a dopamine binge.

This is why pornography causes a vicious circle. When someone views pornography, he gets overstimulated by dopamine; so his brain destroys some dopamine receptors. This makes him feel depleted, so he goes back to pornography, but, having fewer dopamine receptors, this time it requires more to get the same dopamine thrill; but this causes his brain to destroy more receptors; so he feels an even greater need for pornography to stimulate him."

The addict will walk away from porn, head into the bedroom, and there is the female he's already been with hundreds or thousands of times. When he tries to perform sexually with this person, he may have difficulty doing so.

Pornography has become an epidemic among young men. We know pornography warps sexuality, and based on what we know about the brain and the study regarding the Coolidge Effect, it should come as no surprise that in America we have the highest rate in the world of erectile dysfunction in males 18-24 years old. Habitual pornography use affects young men in such a way that a real female they are familiar with doesn't continue to sexually gratify them. They've destroyed their dopamine receptors. They increasingly need more and more dopamine to produce the desired results. Their brain is looking for new, receptive, and willing partners. Real life isn't always moaning and panting and the woman telling the man how amazing they are, but the lower brain doesn't know that. It doesn't differentiate between the women on the screen and the woman they are in a relationship with.

Just a reminder, your sex life isn't what caused him to turn to porn. He most likely already had issues with porn, and his brain has now been wired in a way that he feels like he has to turn to porn to perform. Porn didn't ruin your sex life; your sex life was ruined because of porn.

Josh, the former pornography addict:

Porn ruined your sex life, even if he says it's the other way around. If he blames you at all, it's because he doesn't want to face the shame he feels and the damage his addiction has caused. Odds are, he's done a lot of manipulating of situations as an addict and he just wants to gaslight you into thinking you're part of the problem. You're not. You didn't cause the problem.

If he wasn't already an addict when you met, odds are the seeds had been planted and nothing you did or didn't do in the bedroom had anything to do with his descent into addiction. If the next time you're together you bring two blonde 21-year-old cheerleaders into the bedroom for the orgy he's always wanted, it's not going to cure his addiction. He'll just want three cheerleaders next time and continue to blame you for his completely unrelated problem.

Since masturbation usually accompanies viewing pornography, the viewing session is usually over once orgasm is reached, much like it is when having intercourse with you. Since you're dealing with an addict and not a casual viewer, it's easy to confuse the no-strings-attached release one gets when utilizing pornography as a surrogate for the intimacy one has with a partner. They are actually very different things that meet very different needs, and I think both the addict and the partner confuse them because each scenario ends in orgasm.

Your husband may claim to prefer pornography to you, but what he prefers is having a proven, no-maintenance outlet for stress and anxiety release. The porn doesn't nag, the porn doesn't say no, the porn doesn't judge. Real-life partners do all of those things. Real life partners cause stress. His coping mechanism to deal with stress is porn, but that's only one of the surface reasons he uses. His real issues probably run deeper than even he can understand at this point. I made some of my biggest breakthroughs several years into counseling, so if he says that there's nothing wrong or if he thinks he understands why he's addicted, he probably doesn't have anything close to the full story yet.

Is there anything
I could have done differently?

Tony, the mental health professional:

You're probably running through a lot of clichés in your head, both positive ("You can't control anyone else") and negative ("It takes two to tango"). Or there are a lot of questions, such as: "Was it my fault?" "What did I do wrong to contribute to his addiction?" "Why am I not enough?" "Does he not find me attractive?" "Do I not turn him on?" "If I had had more sex, different sex, etc. would he still have turned to porn?" "If he really loves me, how could he do this?" This is normal. It is also normal for a woman who has just found out about her partner's porn addiction and is herself experiencing betrayal trauma, which has symptoms that are very similar to PTSD, to start second-guessing herself.

The effects pornography addiction have on a relationship are different depending on your situation. There is a difference between a couple who has a strong connection and emotional bond, and a couple who has, aside from the addiction, just grown to be incompatible. I have worked with many couples who are one or the other, and I've worked with some who are both.

Let's put it this way: If you are doing things that aren't conducive to a healthy relationship, for example, having an affair—physically or emotionally—withholding affection, showing a lack of support, failing to effectively communicate, etc., you have contributed certain factors to the deterioration of the relationship. His porn addiction, among other possible elements, is certainly one of the factors that he has contributed to the deterioration. This in no way suggests that you caused him to turn to porn. It's just to illustrate that there are many, countless factors that contribute to the relationship as a whole.

In my practice I see a lot of women who discover, or are finally told, their partner has a pornography addiction and their first thought is to try to reverse-engineer the timeline of their relationship, to go back to the point in time where they think they could have "saved" him. This is an exercise in futility.

If you're asking what you could have done differently to stop his porn addiction, that answer is most likely nothing, especially based on the fact that you weren't aware of what was going on in the relationship. Most women are in shock and wondering if they could have fixed the situation, but if their partner had a different condition, like shingles or chronic fatigue syndrome, would you be asking yourself what you could have done to stop it? While those are different types of conditions than pornography addiction, I hope you see my point. You've never had control of the neurological parts of his mind or the pathways in his brain that have been created by his addiction.

There is a big difference between a couple's failing relationship and an individual's addiction within the relationship. You may have contributed to the former, but you had nothing to do with the latter.

Josh, the former pornography addict:

I understand why you'd want to know the answer to this question, but couldn't you ask this about so many aspects of your life?

Reading between the lines, I think what's being asked here is, "What did I contribute to this?" Nothing that could have avoided it.

You did not create his addiction. My wife had nothing to do with my pornography addiction forming because it happened more than a decade before I met her. Did she ever contribute to times of stress that eventually led to me self-soothing through pornography? Yes. But the issue isn't about her causing me stress, it's about me not having a healthy way to manage that stress.

My wife could feed me greasy fried chicken three meals a day. If I have a heart attack at the dining room table, is it her fault? No. I made the choice to eat the chicken. She didn't force it into my mouth.

Whether it's fried chicken or hardcore pornography, it took me a long time to understand that I cannot blame others for my actions and the consequences of them. He may blame you, but it is only because he doesn't understand this concept. Hopefully someday he will.

Is there anything my wife could have done differently? In years past, I would have tried to scapegoat her, saying she wasn't loving enough, or adventurous sexually, or another lame excuse.

If I had problems with my wife in those areas, those were relationship issues, not addiction issues. It's important that you don't confuse those two things as they are entirely different. What you think is an addiction issue could be about your relationship. Ironically, what he thinks is a relationship issue could be his addiction.

You have found yourself in a situation that was not of your creation. You could have done a lot of things differently, but you would have ended up in the same spot, so stop second-guessing yourself.

Is he like this because I won't do certain things in the bedroom?

Tony, the mental health professional:

It's normal for you to wonder how you contributed to his addiction. Many of your questions will be born of this thought. You're going to try to make sense of his addiction through your own lens. By virtue of picking up this book, you've revealed you are a problem solver, but unfortunately, there are just some problems that were both created and have to be solved by your partner, no matter how much they have negatively affected you.

Oftentimes in my practice I find that when I speak to a man one-on-one, typically before I'm made aware of his addiction, he'll mention that he wishes his wife would do more of the things that he sees on his steady diet of pornography.

When I talk to the wife, she'll usually bring it up as well, explaining how she feels he is constantly pushing the boundaries for things she isn't comfortable with and doesn't want to do—the most common being anal sex and bringing a third woman into the bedroom.

When he mentions scenarios like this, as if they are perfectly normal and reasonable requests, I know right away that he's been deeply entrenched in pornography and has developed a skewed view of what is common and normal in most healthy sexual relationships. In a study that was published in 2016, researchers found that only 5% to 8% of women between 18-and-24 (fair to say the most sexually adventurous and liberal age group) had participated in a three-way, and depending on the study you look at, only 20% to 30% of women under 40 have had anal sex. While there is nothing theoretically wrong with women consensually engaging in these behaviors, they are by far the exception and not the norm.

When the couple comes back together and we begin to talk about the intimate part of their lives, this difference of opinion will surface and she'll say something like, "I don't even know where he gets these ideas."

I'll turn to the guy and he will often shrug and say, "I don't know," as if they were just spur of the moment requests. Having done this work for a long time, I recognize that the things he is asking for are things that a lot of porn addicts ask for in a relationship.

Did he amp-up his pornography use because you wouldn't cross certain boundaries in the bedroom? No, he amped up his use because, as has been previously mentioned (see Coolidge Effect), he has binged on porn enough to have gamed the dopamine system, to have fried some of his neurotransmitters that receive dopamine, leaving him searching for strange, twisted, or bizarre types of porn in order to get that same dopamine rush.

Please remember, you should **NEVER** be forced into anything you're not comfortable with or that crosses lines in your mind. In a healthy relationship where you feel like you can both talk about the true desires of your heart, and where it is done from a place of empathy and understanding, of course it makes sense to explore each other sexually in safe, mutually agreed upon ways. But if he's simply wanting you to "do more" or "try this" and it's purely for him, as if you were simply an object, that needs to be discussed. It is not your fault that the pornography has warped his mind to the point that the commonplace view of sex within a relationship doesn't always excited him anymore.

It is extremely important to know that the kind of activity seen in most pornography does not reflect the healthy version of intimacy and connection I try to help my clients achieve.

Josh, the former pornography addict:

I know a lot of people will disagree with me, just like they disagree with me when I say there's no reason people *MUST* consume alcohol. If somebody is able to handle drinking better than an alcoholic, it doesn't mean it's good behavior to engage in. I believe the same can be said for pornography.

I don't believe that pornography ever makes sense in the realm of a healthy person's sexuality.

Pornography distorts real life. Take a look at the plots of pornographic films. They are ludicrous. Ask a real-life pizza guy if he has sex with his delivery customers as much as pornographic movies make it appear. He'll laugh at you.

The common denominator of all pornography is that it objectifies. It removes the heart, soul and brain of a person and renders them as just a physical object. If he watches enough, the brain can begin to rewire itself to think that way in similar circumstances, such as times of intimacy with you.

He might be perfectly capable of having a swinger lifestyle, but if he's with you and you've made it known you have no interest, he should respect it and leave it at that. A healthy man will not push his partner into sexual situations they are uninterested in pursuing.

The unbridled, raw sexual energy he sees in porn that seems to transport the actors to another ecstasy-laden place doesn't exist. They are actors. They are playing pretend. The brain doesn't always recognize that.

Pornography never gave me a false sense of bravado or confidence that carried over to the bedroom. I was also raised with the idea that no meant no, so if I brought up anything "outside the norm" and she shot it down, I let it go.

He may feel like your sex life is boring, and that may be because the pornography has warped his mind or it may be because he is naturally a more adventurous person with his sexuality than you are. Either way, your belief of what is acceptable bedroom behavior did not drive him further toward pornography.

Since he's addicted to pornography, does this mean he cheated on me?

Tony, the mental health professional:

No, not necessarily, and the data shows that it's not likely that he has. The percentage of people viewing pornography is much larger than the percentage of people who actually have physical affairs. While it could have happened, this is not a conclusion I would advise you to jump to unless you have solid proof.

The work that I do with porn addicts is, for the most part, about an addiction of isolation, usually behind a computer screen. Just because they are getting a thrill off of that screen doesn't always mean that they have progressed and made the leap to outside physical relationships. The isolation part of pornography addiction is pretty significant, as it is an addiction steeped in shame. The shame then leads to feelings of a lack of connection to his life, which leads to isolation and over time (again, please see the Coolidge Effect mentioned earlier in the book) leads to the brain needing more and more porn to try and get the same "feel good" effects.

I've seen studies that confirm this, but I can also tell you anecdotally from the work I've done with men and women that women are far more likely to have a pornography addiction escalate to a situation outside of the relationship.

Whatever this male/female difference in acting out is from, it may be part of what makes you suspect him of having an affair. There's a saying I hear often, that men use love to get sex, and women use sex to get love. Sometimes I feel like, although clichéd, it's true.

You hear jokes about men watching pornography and "fast-forwarding" through the talking scenes. When it comes to pornography, most are not utilizing it for romance or intimacy, whereas the women I've treated for porn addiction often are looking for the kind of emotions they read about in romance novels or see in movies like *Fifty Shades of Gray*. Women are looking for a connection much more blatantly than men and men are often looking for sex purely for a physiological release.

Josh, the former pornography addict:

I don't think there is any specific correlation between fidelity and porn addiction. One doesn't necessarily cause the other. I can tell you that in the first 11 years of my marriage, all while addicted to pornography, I didn't once cheat on my wife in the traditional sense. We can debate if talking to women in chat rooms is cheating, but in the case of a traditional affair, I never went down that road.

This is one of the reasons I don't like being labeled as having a "sex addiction." When people think of the word "sex," they immediately jump to intercourse. I had no interest in pursuing women outside of the computer screen.

In talking with male porn addicts, it's clear to me they use pornography as a coping and soothing mechanism. They are not using it as a substitute for intimacy. I never saw it as a replacement for real intimacy. The only thing that sex with my wife and masturbating with pornography had in common was the physical end result of an orgasm.

Yes, some men start with pornography and move on to having affairs and develop intercourse addictions, but there are also plenty of men with intercourse addictions who have no interest in pornography. Plus, as we all know, there are plenty of men with no addictions whatsoever who still cheat on their partner.

It's impossible to say for sure if he cheated on you, but I don't think it's a conclusion that should be reached or an assumption that should be made.

I'm trying not to judge, I'm really not… but I know I am. How do I not come off as judgmental?

Tony, the mental health professional:

I hope the reasoning behind this question is less about looking like the bad guy and more about your internal mental health of not wanting to be consumed by the hate.

Here's the thing, when you get a bomb like this dropped on you, or when your suspicions turn into your reality, it's more normal to have a major reaction than to have no reaction at all. There really is no script and no wrong or right way to react. What you say or do will have to do with your reaction to the immediate betrayal trauma.

In the short-term you probably shouldn't worry too much about your reaction. You're probably going to very quickly try to make sense of your marriage or relationship going back to Day One.

You have every right to be angry and everybody processes anger a little bit differently. I'll sometimes sit across from a woman who is so spun-up that I don't even try to back her off of her immediate judgment and reaction, because those emotions are so real and so raw that she can't be expected to look at this in a calm, collected manner, yet.

"My marriage was a sham from the beginning and everything he told me was a lie!" This statement, or something similar, is the most common reaction. That may sound judgmental to you, but that's okay. Healthier communication can be worked on later. Right now, though, coming off as judgmental is perfectly normal and you shouldn't beat yourself up about it

I'd even add that if someone didn't come off as judgmental and didn't feel a little bit of heat, I would wonder if they were trying to suppress their emotions, and that isn't healthy or helpful to the situation in the long run. There is going to be a point in the future where you don't want to express that frustration or come across as judgmental, but right now is not the time to worry about that. Have the reaction that comes naturally. There will be time to process and eventually work through all of your thoughts, feelings, and expectations.

Josh, the former pornography addict:

I could tell that my wife was trying not to be too judgmental following my public disclosure, but I also know it is human nature to judge even the most benign situations in everyday life. When something as earth-shaking as a pornography addiction comes to light, it's going to stir a range of emotions. That's to be expected. In fact, I'd worry something were wrong if you weren't affected emotionally.

He's a Porn Addict...Now What?

You're not going to find anybody who thinks pornography addiction is a good thing. Addiction is an illness and robs the addict of certain aspects of their life. Are you feeling some regret over judging an addict because you know he is sick? That's also understandable. When you take a step back from the initial betrayal and divorce your opinion of pornography from the situation, you're left with a person you love who is mentally ill.

I know my wife saw my actions as despicable, but I also know that she wanted me to get better and return to being more like—or even better than—the person she fell in love with so many years earlier. She tried not to be hurtful because it probably would have stunted my recovery, not helped it.

If your friends or family find out about this situation, you'll face some judgment. Everybody in my community found out about my transgressions, and I know my wife felt stupid at times for standing by my side because she was being judged. Reading comments on social media that were inaccurate and nasty was hurtful. She didn't want to turn that hurt back on me.

I think it's okay that she mildly judged me, and I think I deserved it. I believe taking a look at a situation and assessing it is probably a very healthy thing. Had she not judged what had happened and what was happening, I may not have had as successful a recovery. She accurately judged I was a broken man and that I wanted to fix that.

Can a guy really look at pictures and images without comparing them to the person he is with?

Tony, the mental health professional:

I know from working with enough addicts that the typical reason someone is addicted to pornography is that it's a coping mechanism for the parts of their life that they aren't satisfied with and it becomes an addiction they turn to again and again despite the isolation and shame. The pictures in the magazines and the images that they're watching in the videos are an unhealthy escape.

But unfortunately, even when they aren't isolated and are with their wives, they are still preoccupied with the fantasy imagery. A lot of the clients I work with admit they think of pornography when they are intimate with their wives. For young men, the growing rates of erectile dysfunction because of pornography is staggering. They are now growing up with such an unhealthy diet of porn and pictures that they are clearly seeking pixels over people and it shows up in the inability to perform physically because the real person in front of them may not have the perfect body, or may not look as excited to be with them as the women on their computer screens.

Once one jumps into that hole of thinking about pornography while being intimate with their partner, it's difficult for them to get themselves out. I'll sit with a husband and wife in a group session and the man will begin to talk about how often he objectifies women. It doesn't have to be porn. It can just be looking at a woman's breasts instead of her eyes when he's talking, or his eyes going straight to a woman's backside if he passes by them.

I don't think I've met a woman yet who hasn't been absolutely appalled and shocked when she hears how much her husband objectifies women, even in the cases where porn isn't a problem in the relationship. Obviously porn pours gasoline on the fire with the concept of objectification.

Knowing what we know about the way the theater of the mind works, the unfortunate reality is there is most likely some comparison happening. But there is hope! As men recognize their unhealthy relationships with porn and their sexuality, they can truly begin to heal. The first step is bringing awareness to these types of behaviors, like objectification, because they can truly find themselves being aware of looking at a woman and then gently bringing the focus elsewhere.

Josh, the former pornography addict:

I'm sure there are some who can, but if your man is a pornography addict, he's probably not in that rare category.

There are a lot of ways to make comparisons. My guess is that you're wondering if he thought about the women he saw in porn when he was with you. Maybe. Pornography represented a fantasy world of no problems, no responsibility and endless sex with whoever he wanted. You represent the real world of bills, screaming children, making a living, responsibility and sex with the same person for the 1,000th time.

I think the bigger question here is what real harm does that fantasy cause and is it really connected to his porn addiction—or are humans just hardwired for fantasy? You've got enough going on with the real problem of his pornography addiction. His fantasy world should eventually be addressed with a professional, but for the moment, it's not the most pressing issue. It's like rushing to the emergency room with a bullet wound and the nurse pointing out he has a hangnail.

Depending on how you view it, his thinking about being with someone else—whether they were an actor in pornography or just a random person on the street—may be some kind of betrayal or even emotional cheating. If it is a big deal, make note of it so you can address it later, but for now, it shouldn't be among the top priorities. It would have just clouded things for me at the time.

I think I need him more than he needs me. That gives him all the power. Should I just keep quiet?

Tony, the mental health professional:

It's easy to start future-casting and catastrophizing here. It's perfectly normal to think, "If I say something, he's going to flip his lid," or "There's no way this is going to end well. What if it ends in divorce? I don't make enough money to support myself and our children without him. I'm going to end up in an apartment in the bad part of town. I don't want to share custody with him knowing that he views pornography in his spare time. What if the kids were somehow exposed to it? He'll probably get our friends' support. Maybe I should keep quiet because the alternative is not worth the risk. It's just the trade-off I have to endure."

Those feelings of wanting to keep quiet are normal, but ultimately you have to find your voice if you're going to live an authentic life. This is part of the process, and it's always going to feel uncomfortable. That doesn't mean it's wrong. When you are confronted with events that feel scary, when you're not sure what comes next—and in this case, there are a lot of "what ifs" that can feel incredibly heavy—your brain is not only wired to go into fight-or-flight mode, it has a third mode known as freeze. In freeze mode we basically just want to ignore the problem and hope that it will go away. Often your partner is hoping for the same thing at this point. Can we just get back to our regular life?

Your brain is telling you stories that everything is going to work out poorly, but this is where I want to say, "Trust me." This process feels heavy and difficult now, but you're just beginning a series of steps that will bring you to a point where you are going to feel more empowered. Step one is always going to be the scariest, and you're never going to make that step if you're already looking ahead to step 10. Right now, you only have to take step one. Then you move from step one to step two, and then you see what step three feels like.

I don't think that I've ever worked with a woman, either individually or in couples therapy, who didn't say she felt better, more empowered, and as if she were carrying a strength she never had before once she took that first step and allowed the process to play itself out.

Almost always, in bringing up the addiction after healing has occurred, it ultimately helped the relationship. Couples will say, "We hate we had to go through this, but it was for the best. Now we're open and honest and aren't hiding things. Our relationship is stronger and we've discovered that we are...something positive..."

Of course, there are instances when he won't address the problem and refuses to get help. The woman may make the decision to move on, but when this happens, she's moving on as an empowered woman, a woman who is living her truths, being authentic, and ready to start a new chapter not as the woman she was moments after she discovered the pornography addiction.

Josh, the former pornography addict:

No way. There has been a massive shift in your relationship with the revelation of pornography addiction. Things are never going to be the same, and if you sit there quietly stewing in your anger, resentment and sadness, you're going to become an unhealthy person.

When everything came out about my addiction, I don't think it took my wife long to decide that she was going to work to keep the family together. I don't know if it was even actually a decision or a natural instinct. I'm very lucky this way. I've seen families torn apart because the addict is kicked out or the woman leaves and they never have a chance to work out what happened.

My wife put our children first in every situation, as she should. She also put my recovery in front of outward judgment. She never made me grovel for forgiveness. I offered it on my own as I went through the process.

Like she almost always did, she put us before herself. The years leading up to me hitting rock bottom weren't wonderful and our relationship was quite strained, leading to her putting on a lot of weight.

A few months after starting in on my recovery, she did a handful of sessions with a therapist, but for her own mental wellness. She needed to physically feel better. While I was fixing myself, she went through the process of being approved for bariatric surgery and eventually lost over 100 pounds. Now she has a better outlook on life than she ever did.

I know part of her would have liked to bolt, and part of her probably could have stayed stuck in her "take care of everybody else" mode, but she didn't. She recognized that a relationship is not about who has power, it's about communication, shared goals and personal wellness.

Thankfully, neither of us have codependency issues, but I've met enough people through the process to know that it's common in a relationship with an addict. You may want to look into this if you think it's better to stay quiet.

It's not just the addict who gets sick...it's everybody around them. You can't love an addict and be such an important part of their life and vice versa without feeling some effect of the illness. This is where it's important to talk to someone who is a professional.

He says I should accept it because looking at pictures or videos is a better alternative than cheating. Does he have a point?

Tony, the mental health professional:

Yes and no. There's a concept for overcoming addiction called "harm reduction," and in that world, yes, it's better to view porn than cheat, and better to not view porn than view porn, but I worry that at this point, especially after disclosure, if he's saying things like this, he's trying to emotionally manipulate you. This isn't a mathematical formula to be worked out. Some people would view physically cheating as worse, and some wouldn't. Either way, he is turning away from the relationship and robbing the relationship of an intimate connection, and there is no reason to accept that.

I understand when people can say they are honestly not addicted to pornography and are just a casual user, but at the end of the day, there's really nothing beneficial or valuable about viewing pornography—especially from an emotional standpoint.

Pornography affects trust. I think a lot of men and women don't have an idea of what intimacy in their relationship could look like because they've never had it modeled in their life, and they're certainly not going to find it in pornography. Relationships are not built on a foundation of sex; sex should be the byproduct of a healthy relationship.

In a relationship where one or both of the individuals regularly turn to pornography, I believe there is a lack of a deeper connection and more effective tools of communication have not been developed. Anytime there is a need or desire to turn to someone else for a physical or emotional connection—which is exactly what pornography is a substitute for—they are selling themselves short on what their relationship could be. Unfortunately, many just don't have the tools to get there on their own. But there is help...

Josh, the former pornography addict:

Only if you think someone has a point when they say, "Sure you've got a broken leg, but at least we don't have to amputate it!" What he's doing here is classic minimizing and gaslighting.

Manipulation of certain situations and people's thoughts is the currency of the addict. I built a world around me where I believed I was in full control, and when that was challenged, most of the time I could work my manipulative magic and force whoever the squeaky wheel was to get with the program—MY PROGRAM.

Is his addiction to viewing pornography better than physically having relations with somebody other than you? I think most people would say yes. But his addiction to pornography is also better than if he had participated in a school shooting or stolen millions of dollars from elderly people. He can try to compare sins to make you realize things could always be worse, but is that really how you should judge the severity of a situation?

You don't have to accept anything. If he's saying this so he can continue using pornography, you have to ask yourself if that's a breaking point for the relationship. If he's saying this so you'll stop harping on him during recovery, he's still minimizing but at least he's trying. He will hopefully recognize his faulty thinking eventually, just not today.

Letting go of manipulation is a tremendous surrender on an addict's part. Recovery really is all about surrendering a certain way of life. It's scary. That's not an excuse for the addict's behavior up to that point, but I personally know just how hard it is to go from being a manipulative, lying jerk to being someone who strives to live life on Mother Nature's terms.

You need to pay attention to why he's saying something almost as much as what he's saying. Saying that you should accept what he's doing is ludicrous, but more importantly, why doesn't he realize this?

Tony Overbay & Joshua Shea

Chapter 3
Understanding the Addiction

Is porn addiction even a real thing?

Tony, the mental health professional:

In June 2018, the World Health Organization classified "compulsive sexual behavior" as a mental health disorder in their International Classification of Diseases (ICD) list for the first time. While this decision was met with controversy, for mental health professionals and people struggling with pornography addiction (as well as their spouses), it is the closest thing to a diagnosis there has ever been.

The ICD-11 (11th edition) defines compulsive sexual behavior disorder as a "persistent pattern of failure to control intense, repetitive sexual impulses or urges resulting in repetitive sexual behavior."

With that said, I suppose one can call porn addiction a "real thing," but I have never cared much about the debate over whether it is an addiction or not. I've had thousands of people in my office and in my online pornography recovery program over the years who have been unable to stop viewing pornography and masturbating when they have clearly wanted to, even when it has affected their relationships, jobs, and emotional health. At this point the debate of addiction versus not addiction has been somewhat irrelevant to me.

I have people in my office who are looking at pornography and masturbating multiple times a day. They tell me that it's not a major problem, just something they'd like to stop. Conversely, on a couple of occasions I've had men who only look at videos of bikini models, but they can't stop doing it. Who is the addict? Does it matter if there is a diagnosis? Both men want to stop their behaviors. Each of them see the "problem" differently, so if I were to tell the first person he's an addict and the second person that they aren't, there's a chance that the first person would be offended for me judging them or putting them in a box, and the second person may feel like I'm not taking their "truth" or their problem seriously.

I often will say the same thing to both of them. I'm not a big guilt or shame guy, and I'm not one who worries about the label of addiction. The thing they have in common is that they want to put it behind them, but neither can.

I'm grateful that for those who may need a label, we now have one. To me, porn addiction is absolutely a real thing, but I don't think dwelling on labels is what makes people do the work and get better.

Josh, the former pornography addict:

Technically, I guess it depends on who you talk to at any given point in time. When the World Health Organization announced Sexual Impulse Disorder was a diagnosable condition in mid-2018, it was a great move toward the medical community finally accepting it.

When I asked my therapist what she thought about this move toward "legitimizing" porn addiction, she said, "It will only really matter when it's finally a billable option for the insurance companies."

She has a point. Most insurance companies still don't acknowledge gambling addiction as a real condition worthy of coverage, despite the fact it's been widely accepted by the medical community and properly documented as a legitimate addiction. If the insurance companies won't recognize something as an addiction, does that mean it's not a real thing?

I go back to the basic definition of addiction, and that's when somebody is engaging in a certain kind of behavior that they recognize causes negative results and that they wish they could stop, but when push comes to shove, they still engage in.

Many people confuse the words addiction and habit. If you want to learn the difference (and just want to read a terrific book) check out Charles Duhigg's *The Power of Habit*. He clearly explains that a habit comes with a payoff that is positive. Addictions don't.

Ultimately, I think it's up to the individual to decide if they are an addict or if they are witnessing addict behavior. There are some addicts who will never admit it, but clearly fall into that category. You may be in a relationship with one of those.

Is porn addiction a real thing? Does the answer to that really change anything about your situation? I think it absolutely is a real thing based on my experience and the similarities it had with my alcohol addiction.

Could it be used as an excuse for bad behavior? Sure it can, but that doesn't diminish the fact that there are millions of men and women coping with it legitimately.

He says what he's looking at isn't pornography. So, what is pornography?

Tony, the mental health professional:

That's such a great question, and I actually think there's a pretty simple answer. Pornography can be defined as any visual material that one utilizes for sexual gratification.

I've had men come into my office and claim that they don't have a pornography problem because what they use isn't really pornography. They only turn to it for a little excitement. If he is objectifying a person for sexual gratification or stimulation that isn't his wife or partner, there's a deeper issue here, a lack of connection to a partner, or a lack of fulfillment in life. Whatever it is, we need to address the deeper issue.

I had a client who was using hardcore pornography. He thought he could wean himself off of pornography by focusing on the women's faces instead of their naked bodies. But his viewing and masturbating habits continued just the same, only now he was looking into their eyes instead of at their breasts. I had to explain to him that he really hadn't changed anything, because he was still using visual aids for sexual gratification and he was still objectifying the women he was looking at.

This man didn't change his relationship with his sexuality, he just changed the type of pornography he was using to satisfy his desire for sexual stimulation and gratification.

Josh, the former pornography addict:

I read the results of a survey the other day and in the comments section a man said he was first introduced to pornography through HBO. Another said Victoria's Secret catalogs. My first reaction was, "Hey! That's not porn!" But if they think it is, am I really in any position to argue?

Throughout my recovery, my dealings with the law, writing my book and the vast amount of research I've done on the topic in general, I've only seen textbook definitions of the word pornography. I have reached the conclusion that pornography is not a "thing"—it's a concept.

It's a grand idea that can be delineated a hundred different ways. For instance, when I say the word "vehicle," what does that mean to you? We can all agree it has to do with transportation, but our individual definitions lay in the details.

We can probably all agree that pornography involves the depiction of sexual behavior. Most courts won't define it, preferring to use the word "obscenity." Beyond that, it gets tricky.

Since I was a kid, I always associated sex with nudity. I thought there were only three reasons to be nude: A medical examination, taking a shower or having sex. I was raised in a conservative home where people didn't walk around naked. We didn't talk about sex; we didn't display nudity—and my mom's reaction to both were the same—so there had to be a connection.

I think we can agree a strip club has certain sexual connotations. Is it the same thing with a nude beach? Many strip clubs aren't allowed to go bottomless. So, are completely nude people at the beach more sexual because they are displaying their sex organs? Are either of these instances actually pornographic since it's "real life"?

I go back to the survey I read the other day. It was conducted by a Christian group, so I expected more conservatism in the answers, but the men who provided comments really opened my eyes to what some consider pornography. Like the nude beach, Cinemax movie or whips-and-chains scenarios, it caused me to really think about what I mean when I use the term "pornography."

Can I just say, "I know it when I see it"? If some guy thinks a Victoria's Secret catalog is porn, but I think it's more just a nuisance on my end table...who is right? *Penthouse Magazine* is more explicit than *Playboy*, but which one is porn? Both? Neither? Am I indulging in pornography sitting at a strip club, or do I have to be watching on TV or a computer? Does the medium matter? Is it porn if it's real life vs. digital or printed?

I think it comes down to the usage and intent. If I am looking at it for either a sexual rush, as a matter of escapism, a coping mechanism or any other addiction-related reason, then yes, it's pornography. It doesn't necessarily have to be explicit.

What are the odds he can be cured?

Tony, the mental health professional:

"Cured" is another one of those words I don't love, but I do think people can become fully recovered from pornography addiction. The odds he will get better are directly proportional to the amount of work he's willing to do to overcome the addiction. A lot of that will also have to do with how he sees himself. There are people sitting in Alcoholics Anonymous (AA) meetings who have been to three meetings per week for 20 years and still see themselves as being in very active recovery, meaning they say that they are always going to see themselves as an addict.

There are also people who attend 12-step meetings for months, or years, feel like they understand the principles or that the meetings helped them through a rough spot of their lives, and then they stop attending, never drink again and truly believe that alcohol was something from their past. I don't think either way is necessarily right or wrong. If you're able to maintain sobriety, that's the important thing.

I have clients who get progressively better and in doing so, begin to have hope. With this hope they begin to realize they no longer need pornography in their lives. It's also helpful for an addict to take a look at his hypersexuality and begin the process of changing his entire relationship with sex. This usually is a big piece of pornography releasing its mental grip.

I have found that overcoming pornography addiction is truly about embracing life and working as hard as possible to build on the areas where the addict felt less-than, or where they didn't feel like they were in control of their lives, because that is when they turn to pornography. Overcoming pornography addiction is about feeling connected to their spouse or partner, their health, their career, their children, their spirituality; it's about living an authentic life. When people truly embrace the power that they have within them to make positive change in their lives, pornography loses its hold on them.

Josh, the former pornography addict:

This isn't a broken leg, and it isn't the kind of disease that gets cured. If he's actually an addict, he has changed his brain chemistry, and it may not return to pre-addiction condition. Don't think about this in terms of being cured. As I write this, I have been over five-and-a-half years without a relapse, but I know I still have that addict mind.

Instead of worrying about a cure, worry about managing the addiction. First, he's going to have to admit he has an addiction and that he wants to get help for it. Recovery is hard, plain and simple. When I think of the rehab, therapy sessions, 12-step groups, etc. that have been an investment in my recovery, I would guess it's got to be around 10,000 hours. Who knows how many thousands of hours it will be for the rest of my life. Recovery is a commitment.

Many people aren't successful early in making that commitment. I'm rare in that there has never been a relapse. While I do believe relapse is a failure of working a recovery program, I do think it's an opportunity to gather data to make that program stronger moving forward.

If he agrees to attempt recovery, the best thing you can do is support him. Try not to judge if he slips, and try to maintain a safe environment where he feels open to communicate. I speak from experience when I say that it is so much easier and feels so much better to achieve sobriety and maintain a recovery program when your loved ones are behind you.

I don't think I'm ever going to be cured, but I don't think I'm ever going to use pornography again.

Does this mean he was sexually abused as a child?

Tony, the mental health professional:

What we're really talking about is at what point in his life was he sexualized? When did he become aware of his sexuality as well as of those around him? Sexualization is a normal, healthy part of growing up. It is the time that the boy, or girl, begins to see members of the opposite sex (assuming they are heterosexual) in a sexual light—not meaning that they want to engage in sexual intercourse with someone, but that they begin noticing the various parts and pieces of the male and female anatomy and see them in a new light.

Most of us become sexualized during puberty. Our body goes through changes physically and hormonally and we're almost "forced" to deal with our sexuality, as it seems out of our control. As recently as the last decade or two, when a child was sexualized at a younger age, it was primarily thought that they were the victim of molestation or sexual abuse.

Mass media (magazines, television, internet) has changed that assumption. We now know that early exposure to pornography presents many of the same habits in a child as in one who has been sexualized through molestation or sexual abuse.

Let me give you an example. For the average third grader, the woman we call Mrs. Smith, aka "our teacher," comes into the room to teach us each morning. For those who have been sexualized, it's Mrs. Smith who now has breasts who comes into the room. She has curves and cleavage, and someone who has been sexualized is now aware of these parts. This awareness will often cause him to then fantasize about her, while someone sitting next to him who has never been sexualized simply sees her as somebody who is writing on the chalkboard and handing back his schoolwork. In the past, we would assume the child who thought that had some kind of first-person exposure, but now, we know the child may have developed that attitude through viewing pornography. If he was abused, you may not be the first person he wants to talk about it with (if he wants to talk about it at all), as he has most likely been steeped in shame and guilt throughout his life due to the early sexualization.

Josh, the former pornography addict:

Not always, but it can be a sign that there was abuse early in his life.

When I was a child, I experienced abuse at the hands of a non-family member who took care of me prior to entering school and in the afternoons once I began. I witnessed abuse of other children that was far worse than what I remember happening to me. While there was some sexual inappropriateness, the abuse I suffered was more mental, as it's clear to me now this caregiver clearly had mental health issues.

For many, many years, I suppressed the specifics of what happened to me and the other children. When this woman died years ago, I was happy. My mom, who delivered the news, thought I'd be upset, but she could see the joy in my face. I didn't quite understand the joy, I just knew that I didn't like my experience there.

It wasn't until I started working one-on-one with a sex therapist when I was seeking treatment for my alcoholism at a California rehab that the memories started flooding back. He helped me remember more than a dozen incidents of abuse. If I had not worked with this therapist, I don't know if I would have tapped into these memories.

More important than remembering the individual moments was working to understand what they meant to me at the time and how they helped shape me as a person, especially when it came to coping mechanisms and survival skills. Much of who I was as a person—the kind of person who could hugely overachieve while at the same time hiding alcohol and porn addiction for two decades—can be traced back to that experience, for good or bad.

There are people who can go through traumatic situations and it has no connection to later addiction. I believe that what happened to me under that caregiver's watch played a giant part in my later problems. It wasn't the only thing, but it was a major part.

He may have been abused and not remember. He may have been abused and not want to talk about it. He may not have been abused. It's an important topic, though, and it's one that he should talk about with a professional.

One of the biggest keys to my recovery was going through the experience of remembering and analyzing this abuse. Statistics suggest that most addicts, regardless of substance, have some kind of trauma or abuse in their past, and porn addiction is no different.

If he's an alcoholic or gambling addict, is he more likely to be a porn addict?

Tony, the mental health professional:

More likely? Yes, but don't mistake that answer for me saying that he most certainly MUST be a porn addict. My comments are based on the concept of addiction in general. Primarily, that addictions come from feeling "less than" or not-connected to a spouse, children, a career, health, faith, or any of those areas. When someone feels discomfort in any of those areas, the brain wants to avoid the discomfort by turning toward an addiction, any addiction.

Addiction has triggers such as anger, loneliness, hunger, or being tired. They will often manifest in real life events, like a bad day at work. With addiction, his brain is now conditioned to turn to whatever will give him that jolt to the pleasure and reward centers of the brain. It can be fed by drugs, gambling, video games, food and yes, pornography.

If you think about it, pornography is one of the easier things to become addicted to in our world. If you want alcohol, you have to go out and buy a bottle. If you want to play blackjack, you have to find a casino. Pornography is low-hanging fruit considering the ease with which it is delivered via the internet and social media apps. If one addiction makes the pain go away, having two addictions gives you options for making the pain dissipate. I would guess that over half of my male clients are addicted to something in addition to their pornography, often something that is more socially acceptable, like gambling or drinking, or even exercising or working.

Josh, the former pornography addict:

If someone is any kind of addict, they do run a higher risk of being addicted to another substance or behavior. More importantly, if your husband or boyfriend doesn't seem to be an addict and is very new to recovery, he's in the sweet spot for cross-addiction to occur.

I had addict behavior my entire life. Even as I was living with my pornography and alcoholism, it was not hard to get addicted to something else and create a triumvirate. I think one of the things that did me in over the final three active years of my addictions was that work became an addiction with just as strong a pull—and that did just as much damage—as the old standby addictions mustered.

I heard the message in both of my rehabs that early recovery can be a dangerous time for a person, because they can be getting free of one substance and feeling a sense of accomplishment while not recognizing they are in the early stages of addiction with another.

If your partner is a porn addict and seems to be doing a good job, but is now playing poker with his buddies twice a week and wants to visit the nearby casino every weekend, there may be a problem developing there. He could be just trading an old addiction for a new one. That's not recovery.

The "high" he got from the porn is being replaced by the high of that perfect hand in Texas Hold 'Em or hitting three Double Diamond symbols in a row on a slot machine.

In my life now, I am very vigilant about not developing new addictions, even with the work I do around porn addiction education. There are days that I could appear on three podcasts and create another blog posting. Those are good things, right? Only if they're not interfering with the time I spend with my wife and kids or one of the freelance writing projects I need to make money.

Addicts know the great feeling they get from their addiction when things go well. When you hit 21 in Blackjack or find that perfect pornographic film clip, the dopamine floods the brain. Now that they are not allowed to get that rush with a certain behavior, it's almost understandable they'd look for it another way.

Odds are, you find gambling less morally objectionable than pornography. It would probably be easier for him to develop an addiction you don't have as much against as pornography. Be aware that this could be happening. The excuse, "At least it's not porn, right?" will only lead to other problems later on.

Is it easier for a younger man to beat porn addiction than an older one?

Tony, the mental health professional:

That's an interesting question because I think there are a couple of things at play. When I have younger men in my office and we begin to talk about what recovery may look like, they will tell me so many more times than older men, "I can do this on my own."

I also find that younger men are much less willing than older ones to do the work that it's going to take to get deep into recovery, meaning making large changes in their lives and embracing the uncomfortable feelings that they may have in their relationships, careers, parenting, or health. They may feel that taking up a daily mindfulness practice isn't necessary, or attending group meetings, or having an accountability partner, or installing a monitoring app on their computers or phones, or allowing their spouse access to their social media accounts. "This time," they'll typically say, "I'll be more serious about stopping!" Only they've been telling themselves that for years, if not decades.

Of course I'm generalizing here, but young men seem to think pornography addiction is not a big deal and there is an easy fix, like, "If I only had more sex in my life or I was in a relationship, this wouldn't really be a problem."

My older clients typically don't say the same thing. They recognize what a giant chunk of their life has been taken by porn addiction and the damage that it's caused, so they're ready to do whatever it's going to take to put this behind them.

Put in simple terms, over time habitual patterns of both behavior and thought become filed away into the "habit center," or the part of the brain called the basal ganglia. The brain wants to be lazy. It believes that if it doesn't have to do too much work it will live for a long time. When a pattern of behavior or thought becomes a habit, the brain goes into au-topilot when triggered. So, if a trigger is feeling dissatisfied in one's work, the brain will say, "Hey, I got this one. He wants to look at pornography and masturbate. We'll take it from here!" When he feels like he's a crummy parent and his wife doesn't appreciate him, again, the brain says, "Okay, we're on it. Let's get him numbing out to some porn."

If you look at the way the brain works and the deep patterns of behavior that have taken place from years, or decades, of giving in to the addiction, on a physical level it may be more difficult to reverse the entrenched patterns of behavior, but it's certainly not impossible. The addict must have hope in order to overcome this addiction, and that hope starts with them acknowledging the problem, being aware of how difficult it has been for them to overcome, and being aware of the work that lies ahead of them.

I will say that I have worked with hundreds and hundreds of men who have, in fact, overcome their addiction to pornography and masturbation, and they find themselves in better relationships, with better health, and more in tune with their spirituality and their careers. Regardless of how long they have been addicted to porn, they can begin to reverse porn's negative effects.

Josh, the former pornography addict:

And now, you've run into the wall that I have run into many times as I seek to educate myself about pornography addiction. Hopefully there is a researcher sitting at a university somewhere in this world pouring over anonymous questionnaires given to recovering porn addicts who will produce a report about the correlation between age of recovery and success. At the time I'm writing this, there is no such report.

I thought if I could find reports that talked about the age of successful recovery in other genres of addiction, there may be a way to extrapolate data, but it appears researchers are more interested in studying what causes drug addiction or alcoholism than what fixes it.

In the various rehabs, group therapy and 12-step rooms I've been in, I can report what I've seen, and it's that older people seem to take their recovery more seriously.

When I've seen a judge order someone to rehab, it's usually someone under 35. That's also the same age group that gets forced into rehab by Mommy and Daddy at the threat of getting cut-off from the money stream.

Much like there is no stereotype for your average addict, I'd say there's no stereotype for your average person in recovery. Older people can use the excuse, "I've been this way forever, so I can't change now," while younger people can think, "I have my whole life ahead of me. I better fix this now." Recovery seems as much about self-motivation as anything else, and that's not native to one demographic.

I think it has so much less to do with the age than the quality of the recovery. If your partner thinks a decades-long pornography addiction can be fixed with a once-a-week trip to Sex Addicts Anonymous, I'll put my money on the 22-year-old who went to an inpatient treatment center.

I don't know if I would have succeeded to the point I have now if I tried recovery at 25. Aside from unlikely being able to embrace the idea I was an addict, I probably would have treated the whole thing as a joke because I didn't have much to lose. My career hadn't been established, and aside from a car payment, I had yet to learn what real responsibility was.

With a wife, two kids, two car payments, a mortgage, the need to re-establish myself professionally to earn money and the other trappings of adulthood, I took recovery seriously and the results are clear.

Don't worry about if he's young or old. His attitude is what is going to make him succeed or fail.

I can understand how somebody gets addicted to drug or alcohol, but porn should be easier to quit. Why won't he just stop?

Tony, the mental health professional:

I think this question shows a little bit of naivete on behalf of the non-addict. You may not be addicted and you may have just found out about the addiction, but you're talking about years of behavior that led up to where he is right now. You may only be looking at the tip of the iceberg, and as any boat captain can tell you, it's not the ice on top of the water you have to be worried about, it's what is hiding under the surface. Recovery is the work of drilling through that iceberg and seeing just how many miles under the surface of the water it goes.

I had a client who was a very successful man and he ended up losing his wife because he just couldn't get his porn addiction in check. She was beautiful, they had a great family and he made more money than I'll ever see, but he couldn't let the porn go. I remember he once said to me, "I wish I was addicted to alcohol or cocaine, because then I could just not buy it. How am I supposed to quit when my addiction is in my pocket on my phone? Yeah, I could put filters on everything and try to block it, but I've got so much stored up in my brain that I can work with."

I think that illustrates just how deep this addiction can run. They've been separated a few years now, and while the addiction doesn't affect his professional life that I'm aware of, it clearly demolished his personal life.

I think he's incorrect in believing the "grass is greener" with a different addiction, but that's the mindset of an addict: "If I only hadn't become addicted to *THIS*!" There isn't any chart or any ranking of addictions of which is easier or harder to recover from that I'm aware of, but even if there were one, does it matter? Pornography addiction is what you're dealing with, and it's serious.

Josh, the former pornography addict:

I think what you're expressing in that question is the belief that society has long held when it comes to addictions.

When I was in rehab in California for alcoholism, a lot of the younger addicts would come through the door with their main addiction being heroin or meth. Almost always, once they started talking, it was clear they also had an issue with alcohol.

Eventually, when they got comfortable, they'd almost inevitably say something to the effect of, "You're lucky. You're only addicted to alcohol, but I have something much worse."

It was slightly insulting, but I understood where they were coming from. We rank our addictions in society, and since porn addiction is still so new to the mainstream, it ranks somewhere around video game addiction as something to take seriously.

When it came to the alcohol, I had to point out to them that they couldn't walk into any 7-11 and get heroin or meth, but I could get my drug of choice. When I went out for a nice dinner with my wife, my drug of choice has its own menu known as the Wine List. Perhaps their drug could ravage their body quicker, but mine was legal, and it was everywhere.

If porn is what your partner is addicted to, it's going to be the most difficult thing in the world to quit, and comparing him to somebody else who had a different addiction altogether isn't fair to him and is just going to frustrate you.

Porn addiction isn't about sex. It isn't about pretty girls. They are just vessels to get at what it's really about, and that's the same thing for every addict, regardless of substance. It's escape.

Imagine if you had to hide the one thing that gave you a moment of respite from the trials of this world, then imagine it stopped working, but you couldn't stop using it.

While cravings and urges with my alcoholism are different than the porn addiction, I put them on the exact same level when it comes to challenges in early recovery and with maintaining my sobriety.

It's not easy to quit. He's an addict, after all.

Chapter 4
My Family and Our Safety

Should I leave him and take the children?

Tony, the mental health professional:

I urge you to get your feet underneath you before you make any significant decisions. When many women first learn of their husband's betrayal, they go into a state of shock. The "fight or flight" mechanisms of the brain kick, adrenaline floods the brain, cortisol, a natural hormone in the body, is released. Cortisol is designed to help you respond to stress or danger. It can be difficult to make rational decisions. I'm guessing that by the time you got this book, you may have had some distance from the initial shock of disclosure or discovery, but there is still a good chance that when you think of the situation, you're triggered. It may be difficult to know what to do.

I recommend running through a checklist in your mind: Are you leaving, or asking him to leave, simply to hurt him? Or do you truly need some space in order to figure out your next steps? Be honest with yourself. Are you trying to make him feel what you are feeling? I don't say this from a judgmental place, but simply from an awareness standpoint. If so, that is a perfectly normal response, but right now you need to do what is best for you, and your kids.

With that said, if you are in a relationship that has experienced moments of emotional or physical abuse, you and your children's safety is of utmost importance. When in doubt, I recommend doing whatever you feel is necessary to be able to process the information that you have heard. Reach out to a therapist, your parents, a clergy member, or someone who you trust who can help you process the information.

If you think that you're going to leave and take the children, where are you going? Do you count on him for financial support, transportation, etc.? What if those things suddenly disappear?

Obviously, this is all a moot point if you believe he is potentially dangerous or could be violent. You need a legitimate safety plan in that case.

Taking your kids away is something that isn't easily forgotten if you end up patching things up, unless the kids won't remember because they are too young.

The last thing you want to do is use your child as a chip in a game of "Who Can Hurt the Other." It's my experience that even in the worst situations, both parties can agree they want what's best for the children, and that is rarely plucking them away from a parent, even if you have major issues with that parent. It's not about the kids, so don't use them as a tool for bargaining.

I do want to caution that there have been many times I've sat in my office and heard a woman who is very upset swear she's not using her kids for leverage. They honestly don't see that they're doing it. Before you do, take a deep breath and try to figure out what's best for the family as a whole.

Josh, the former pornography addict:

Thankfully, my wife didn't leave and never tried to turn the kids against me, so it's hard for me to suggest anything that would disrupt things for you. Since you know your situation—and the best thing could potentially be to leave—I'd just advise you to think carefully about your next move, as it could have lifelong implications for everybody involved.

First and foremost, are your kids safe? In my situation, they had no idea. They were never exposed to the material I looked at and were either not home or fast asleep upstairs when I did. Like most addicts, I was great at hiding things—and this is potentially one of the few times that skill can be a plus.

Second, what will the environment be moving forward? I had such a public humiliation based on my actions that I believe my wife's reaction was to try and hold things together and keep things as normal as possible. There was so much drama swirling around that home was actually one of the few safe places for all of us. You probably have far less drama, and if the kids don't know about what's going on, is uprooting them the best choice?

Aside from the kids, you have to do what is best for you. The children are more resilient than you think. Half the kids in the United States have had to deal with the divorce of their parents over a multitude of issues. Sure, it feels bigger when it's happening to you, but the kids should not be the only consideration of if you stay or go.

Can you still be an effective mother and live with this man while you sort through what his addiction will mean to your future together? Is the environment going to be one where the kids will be exposed to some kind of potential mental, emotional or physical damage if you all stay? In that case, without question, you should go.

How much do we tell the kids?

Tony, the mental health professional:

There is no simple answer to this question. There are as many experts that believe you should tell your children, under the veil of complete family transparency, as there are who believe that the children should absolutely NOT know about a partner's extramarital affair or pornography use. In my practice, I've seen both sides and I've seen them both go well, and I've seen them both unfortunately not.

My first impression, without knowing more about the details of a situation is no, you don't tell the kids. Let the dust settle. If your child is the one who caught their dad on the computer watching graphic pornography then yes, you need to be able to explain what happened and what they saw, and that needs to happen without shaming the child.

However, as with the majority of answers given in this book, there is no exact science to this answer because every child processes information through their own lens, just as we do. One 10-year-old may be able to understand the situation better than another 15-year-old. While there are definitely age-appropriate guidelines, you know your kids better than anyone else, so ultimately use this information as a guide and then adjust per the needs and makeup of each child.

Developmental biologist Jean Piaget is known for developing a blueprint that breaks down the stages of "normal intellectual development, from infant through adulthood." This includes thought, judgment, and knowledge. These stages are Sensorimotor, from birth through approximately 2 years; Preoperational, from toddlerhood, or 2 years, through early childhood (roughly age 7); concrete operational, or roughly ages 7 through 12, and then formal operational, from adolescence through adulthood.

Working from Piaget's model, I find that when it comes to younger children up through early adolescence, unless they were exposed to images or videos or if they were brought around the affair partner and they felt uncomfortable, you don't need to tell the kids. I've processed situations like, "Why was daddy in the bed with that lady from the school?" In situations where they have been exposed, I recommend seeking professional help for the children to learn how best to communicate. The key is that you don't want to ignore questions by your child.

As the kids get older, mid-to-late adolescence to teens, they typically can pick up on problems between parents. I've talked with kids who have told me, "Something is going on and either they think I'm an idiot for not noticing, or they're idiots because they can't see it's happening."

You don't have to get into great detail, but can say something like, "Your father is going through some rough times and I'm trying to support him, but it's a rough time for both of us."

If they press for details, you can let them know it's a private matter, and again, seek help from a professional to help them process as well.

For adult children, especially if they're not living at home, it's a matter of what you want to tell them. I'd leave that up as a group decision between your partner and yourself.

The most important thing is that this information not be used as a weapon against your spouse. You need to keep in mind that you're ultimately trying to work toward what is best for the kids.

Knowing how the kids are going to respond is important, and I've seen situations where a mother knew the kids would immediately vilify the father and she used that as a threat against him. Keep the question, "Why am I sharing any details with my children?" top of mind, and let that answer guide you.

Josh, the former pornography addict:

We had no choice because of the public way I was outed as a pornography addict, since the media reported on it almost immediately. The kids were going to find out sooner than later if we didn't address the situation as it happened. I simply left it at, "Daddy looked at pictures he shouldn't have looked at."

That seemed to be enough of an explanation for my son, and I know my daughter and wife had a deeper conversation about why people look at pornography in which I did not participate. My daughter was 13 at the time and my son was 10.

They didn't seem to care too much about the addiction, but it was more about how it would change our lives. Since I lost my job, they were worried about how we would pay our bills. There was some talk about leaving our town, which hit them both hard. Not surprisingly, like kids do, they made it about how it would affect them, and we made sure to parent them with that in mind.

How open are you with your children about the other issues in your life? If you try to hide money trouble or drama in the family from them, you're probably better off to handle it that way, especially in an age-appropriate context. If your children are older and will probably figure things out sooner or later, you may want to have a conversation with your partner about how to address it. You have one chance to control the situation in relation to your children, and that's at the very beginning.

My first book came out when my daughter was 18 and my son was 15. It got into the reasons I developed, and nurtured, the addiction. My daughter didn't want to read it and my son read the entire thing the day it was released. He said it made him sad in places, but he could handle it. It's out there if she ever wants to get read it, but I'm never going to force her.

If you have older children, or adult children away from home, I think that it comes down to whether you are staying or not. If you are staying, think long and hard before sharing the information about dad's addiction early in his recovery. If you're leaving, you can gloss over it in the short-term and evaluate down the road if it's your place, or his, to say anything.

The family suddenly feels broken. Where does this leave us?

Tony, the mental health professional:

You are going to have a lot of feelings hitting you from all angles and at all times, day and night. You may have moments where you feel like this will make you stronger! Then, within a few minutes, you may feel like you never want to see him again and that a quick punch to his neck is inevitable if you see him in the next few minutes. This is NORMAL. You are not going crazy. Your brain is trying desperately to make sense of things. Your brain is working faster than you even realize trying to process all of the information, and triggers, coming in.

Step back, and give the dust time to settle. Try and bring your family closer. It doesn't have to feel like every meal or every interaction is group therapy time, or time to teach a life lesson. Sit together and watch a movie. Play a board game. Your children may want more time on their own or with their friends. You may need to give them that time. Don't shame them, but do all that you can to try and spend time together.

This is usually the part where the woman is going through the relationship in her mind, not just wondering how she missed the signs, but wondering what else she's missed the signs of, aside from pornography addiction.

I've had women who told me they went all the way back to the first date and are now questioning what is or isn't a lie. Quite often I hear, "I don't know what's real or what to believe."

Don't try to deny the trauma and put on a happy face. It's going to feel like things are out of control and hopeless. Pretending nothing happened isn't going to work right now and it's important to recognize that these are the typical emotions and thoughts of someone in your situation. It's okay to be angry one moment and sad the next. You're really at a fork in the road here, with only a few major options. My suggestion is to get help with the assistance of a professional.

I have sat through literally hundreds of couples going through a similar thing, and while it's hard to believe, this can actually make the relationship stronger. I've seen men decide that now is that time for total honesty in the relationship, and it doesn't take many sessions before communication begins to improve.

Think about what it would be like to be more united in the relationship and how wonderful that would be. If he's on board, you can get there and be stronger than you ever were prior to the disclosure.

Josh, the former pornography addict:

I think that's natural. The very foundation of what it means to be a family is challenged when somebody is found to have an addiction. You can't even pretend that you're living the idyllic family life with the two kids, a dog and a white picket fence anymore. Scratching your head while wondering what the new reality will be like is understandable.

A lot of the answer to this question will have to do with your immediate actions—and his—following the revelation of porn addiction. If you leave, there are a set of questions to answer and actions to be undertaken. If you stay, it's a different set, and no two people are going to have the same situation to evaluate.

In our case, since my wife didn't take the kids and leave, we took a measured, "wait-and-see what happens," approach. About 10 days after I was publicly outed and the media ran with my story, I entered an inpatient rehabilitation facility on the other side of the country. It left me with valuable time to process what the family meant to me, but it also gave them time to heal as a unit.

Here's the great irony of the whole thing: Despite all of the drama, I think I pulled enough of myself together to finally be some level of the father and husband I should have been a lot earlier in our lives together. When that happened, the family actually started to seem healthier as a unit.

As I write this, we're more than five years past the initial fallout. I don't think we're that different than most families at this point. It was a very, very rough patch that could have taken us out, but we all stuck together and ended up better for it on the other side.

His addiction doesn't have to be all doom and gloom. If he's successful in recovery, your lives together may actually become better than either of you could imagine.

What does it mean to create boundaries?

Tony, the mental health professional:

Personal boundaries are a very important part of re-establishing emotional and physical limits in order to protect ourselves from being manipulated, both emotionally and physically, by others. Strong boundaries will not only protect you, but they will begin to empower you. Boundaries can come in many ways, from, "I need you to ring the doorbell before coming in the home," especially if he has temporarily moved out while you are working on things, to, "When you raise your voice at me or make excuses, I am going to disengage from the conversation."

A boundary can be whatever you feel that you need to begin to heal. I remember early in my practice a couple came into my office and the husband had admitted to an extramarital affair. At that point he said that he needed his wife to "back off" because he had said he was sorry and she needed to let him "do his thing." His wife was asking that she be able to see his texts and his emails and that she needed to begin to rebuild trust. He said, "Absolutely not. You just need to trust me now because I told you I was having an affair and I stopped!"

He eventually was caught having another affair, and the red flags had been there all along. I remember that shortly after seeing that couple another couple presented with almost identical circumstances. Only this time something was very different about their interactions. She said she didn't know how she could ever trust her husband again. He said that he understood that, and he said that she could do anything or ask anything of him and he was willing to do it. If she wanted to have every password he owned, if she wanted to see his texts and phone calls, if she wanted him to call every 30 minutes, if she wanted to ride along with him to sales calls, he didn't care. He wanted to respect whatever boundary she set.

Boundaries are about creating space. It's okay for you to want and demand certain things from your partner that you need to see done in order to move forward with the partnership. In most relationships there is a fair amount of give and take, but with a boundary, there is no gray area; it's black and white.

It's okay for you to create that space. It's okay for you to say, "I need to see you doing work. I need to see you going to recovery meetings. I need you not to beg me to come home, and I need you to respect my privacy right now." You have a right to all of those things and anything else that you want (within reason, of course).

What I'll often see happen when a woman creates boundaries for her partner is he tries to minimize the need for them. He's been outed with disclosure and then when she is creating boundaries, he is acting like they are a set of suggestions and not new rules. This is the point where she needs to assert she is allowed to have these boundaries and they are necessary if there is a chance at them moving forward as a couple.

The trickiest part for the woman is holding her ground when the man starts to push back against her boundaries. Before you set a boundary, you have to be determined that there is a cause-and-effect if he break that boundary. She has to be willing to say, "I'm going to leave you if you break my boundaries."

If you set boundaries, you'll probably have to remind him of them repeatedly, and it may not be because he wants to intentionally disobey you. Whether it's conscious or subconscious, a lot of times he'll just continue in his typical pattern of behavior. You can't let this pattern continue.

I've had plenty of times in my office where there has been a disclosure and then we will spend a session or two establishing boundaries, but come the sixth or seventh session, they've all been broken and they'll say, "We're good again." He's good again, and he's probably gaslighted her into believing she is, too.

I've had women actually say to me, "This is just who he is, and I should be grateful for what I have." That breaks my heart because it reveals a level of codependency on her part that is only going to get in the way of healing and recovery. I see many women with codependency issues that only become clear when she tries to create boundaries.

Josh, the former pornography addict:

When I think of boundaries, I think of the edges of a soccer or football field or the spot where one state or country becomes another. I understand the concept of creating boundaries, but they don't always sound serious. After all, what happens if you kick the ball out of bounds in soccer? You just throw it back in and keep going.

As an addict, I get the message more when it's called, "Drawing a line in the sand." I was first introduced to this idea watching a Bugs Bunny cartoon as a kid when Yosemite Sam dragged his heel across the ground and threatened to shoot if Bugs Bunny crossed the line.

Consider yourself Yosemite Sam. You need to draw some very clear lines and explain to your partner that he may not cross them. Do you find looking at porn 100% unacceptable? Tell him. Do you refuse to have a computer in the house moving forward? Tell him. Do you expect him to go get help for his addiction? Tell him.

Then, after you've told him, you have to tell him what happens if he doesn't comply with your demands. Will you leave? Will you seek a divorce? Will you kick him out? He needs to know the consequences of his actions.

Now here's the part when you don't want to be like Yosemite Sam. Bugs Bunny crossed the line. Yosemite Sam didn't shoot. He drew another line. Bugs Bunny crossed that one. Another line, another cross. Another line, another cross.

Bugs Bunny quickly learned—as your husband or boyfriend will—that the lines mean nothing if he can cross them and there are no repercussions. He's been crossing lines with you for a long time. It's just more blatant now that you've created these expectations.

Not only is this important for your mental health, I think it's important for his recovery. If you expect him home for dinner or else call, tell him. It's probably not something to leave over if he doesn't follow it, but it will be a sign of how things are going.

I never felt like my life had consequences. If I had, there was no way I would have ended up talking to a teenage girl online. I was able to talk, charm, negotiate and manipulate my way out of every negative situation—until that day.

My life is full of consequences now, and my wife has created boundaries/lines-in-the-sand that I find neither overbearing nor hard to comply with. I also have boundaries where I didn't before and I'm healthier for it. I think boundaries are one of the first steps when it comes to self-care.

Should I tell other people in his family and see if they can help?

Tony, the mental health professional:

My immediate response is no because typically this is done either from a place of anger or from a place of really meaning well, but not thinking it through. This is something that the two of you are dealing with and bringing in more people can only complicate things, especially if you're not both on board with bringing them in.

If he's getting help and you want to have somebody you can turn to as a confidant, be it a therapist or a spiritual adviser you can confide in, that's fine, but it doesn't mean you get to air all of his dirty laundry to his family.

If the addict is seeking help, or even if they're not, it should almost always be left up to them if they want to talk with their friend, or father, or brother.

Another word of advice: Despite what you may see on television, interventions don't often go well. It's been proven that the whole "get the family together to read their ultimatum letters" thing is not nearly as effective as Hollywood would have you believe. If he's being outed, he's just going to see those letters as threats.

I've had women who, in therapy with me either by themselves or with their husbands say, "We've tried 12-step meetings, we've tried rehab, we've kept it from the kids and I'm working with him as much as I can. He said he wanted more sex, so I gave him more sex. I'll do anything he wants but nothing is working. I think I should talk to his family, right?"

My response is still no.

The only time that I would get his family involved without his consent is if he poses a legitimate safety issue to you or your children.

I think this also holds true for your friends, his friends and those you share together. There was an old children's television show from the 1950s called *Howdy Doody*, and the children who sat in the audience were called "The Peanut Gallery." When Howdy Doody asked for a response to a question, The Peanut Gallery yelled back at him.

I think that all of these other people in your life are like The Peanut Gallery. You're not going to find a family member or friend who simply listens, supports and doesn't share the reality of your situation with someone else.

Your friends are going to want to say the things they assume you want to hear like, "Get rid of him," or, "You deserve better!" You're going to get a lot of advice that tells you just to burn your whole life to the ground and start over. It's my experience that they will also share your plight with other people.

I understand and appreciate the need for a confidante, but it needs to be someone you can 100% trust, like a therapist or spiritual advisor. It's pretty rare when a friend doesn't tell somebody else, and that only makes the situation worse.

Finally, keep in mind that his family is just that: HIS family. Despite delivering shocking news that doesn't paint him in the best light, they have the blood connection to him, not you.

Keep it between the two of you, and let him decide who else may learn of his addiction.

Josh, the former pornography addict:

This is another tough one there is no easy answer for. In my case, when my story hit the media, everybody knew about my addiction overnight: family, friends, neighbors and even people who had no idea who I was.

I was in and out of therapy for years in my 20s and early 30s, yet never once mentioned my porn addiction. I was married for a dozen years and it was never addressed. Short of being publicly outed, I can't fathom a scenario where I would have sought the help of anybody.

Why? Because it's about sex. It's about naked people. It's about what turns you on, which may be kinkier than most or socially frowned upon. It's about a behavior most people pretend they don't engage in. People won't admit to looking at pornography despite statistics proving the vast majority of them do, so how can somebody openly admit to having a problem with it?

The day after I was arrested and my lawyer asked me (with my wife and father in the room) if I had any addictions, I immediately admitted to my alcoholism, which they both suspected. It took me another six months before I stopped blaming the alcohol for the mistake I made.

Looking back now, I don't think I would have progressed to the point that I'm now at in recovery if not for my family. They have been a non-judgmental safe haven in a world where many either don't view pornography addiction as a "real thing" or condemn those who suffer with it.

I believe this question can best be answered by looking at his relationship with his family, looking at the history of the values, opinions and behaviors of his family and if they are open to being part of the process of recovery.

I know how helpful my family has been, but I have talked with so many people where their family's intervention had a different outcome.

Support doesn't mean his mother or sister sitting down and working out with him why he became the way he is. It can be as simple as just letting him know that they love him and have faith he can overcome his addiction. It's about love and support.

If you make the decision to seek help from his family, I would start with the male relative he is closest to and allow them to have input on if, and how, the family should be involved. They may have insight about the family you don't possess.

In the end, I never would have asked my family for help unless it was forced upon me. Thank God that happened.

Chapter 5
The Spiritual Questions

Should I make him tell our pastor?

Tony, the mental health professional:

Remembering that ultimately you can't "make" him do anything, I feel that it is reasonable to ask him to confess to your pastor, especially if he has truly been living a "double life" with regard to the addiction. Many addicts attend church regularly, which can confuse a spouse. "How can he worship God, or teach a Sunday School class, or hold any type of church responsibility and be acting out?" These are hard questions to process for the betrayed, but to the betrayer, this has been part of the shame cycle that often keeps an addict turning back to the addiction.

Many addicts tell me that when they are in church, they are trying to be "all in." They often say that they truly do compartmentalize areas of their lives, and when it comes to church, they often desperately cling to the hope that while they are in their "spiritual compartment" they will feel some hope. Often they are hoping that with enough spirituality they can overcome the addiction.

Unfortunately, however, this actually can feed the addiction. When they are not actively seeking treatment, attending church and then relapsing afterward, whether it be the same day or within a week or a month, regardless of the timeframe, this feeds into their "what's wrong with me" story. They often feel like even though they are going to church, and they feel like that is the correct thing to do and they have spiritual experiences, they must be extremely broken if they continue to turn back to pornography.

I believe that truly turning away from the addiction requires confession to a pastor or other religious leader. However, and this is extremely important, I believe that you need to feel love, or hope, from a pastor in order for the confession to be beneficial. Too often untrained pastors, even therapists, feel like they need to sprinkle a small amount, or worst case a giant bucket full, of shame when the addict comes into their office. This only feeds the addiction. It is imperative for the pastor to let the person know that they are loved, that the pastor is glad they came in, and that they are on the path to recovery together.

I recorded a podcast on this topic that I believe will help both the betrayed and the betrayer on the effects of shame with addiction. I would recommend that you go to my website, find the episode on *The Bishop's Strongest Tools to Help Addicts*, and listen. Tell your pastor that you would like for them to listen before they meet with you.

I feel that it is important to share that I am an active member in the Church of Jesus Christ of Latter-day Saints. The pornography problem in my church is as rampant, if not moreso, than any other faith community. I believe a lot of the reason why this is the case is because of the shame that is felt in a faith community. Well-intentioned leaders often give sermons on the dangers of pornography, which is true, but often those sermons come with the warnings of what will happen to the addict, their marriage, their relationship with their kids, and their relationship with God if they continue in their addiction. Wives often turn to their husbands and say,

"I better not ever catch you doing that!" which leads to more seclusion and isolation with the addiction.

My personal belief is that addictions come from a void in one's life. I find that when a person is not feeling connected to their partner, their kids, their work, their health or their faith, they will often turn to an addiction to numb themselves out of their discomfort. So, an addict truly needs to find their place in their faith community.

Josh, the former pornography addict:

I think you could suggest it, but I don't think you should make him do anything he doesn't want to do. You'll only create resentment that way. If he behaves in a way you don't agree with and makes choices you don't want to tolerate, there's a series of choices you can make. Forcing him to fit your mold will likely not work in the long run.

I would make the suggestion and then step back. I look back at the series of priests that led the churches I belonged to years ago when I lived with my parents, and there was only one I would have felt comfortable enough talking to about this situation.

While most pastors do have experience talking to people in stressful situations, they don't have the kind of training a therapist would have in dealing with this kind of problem. If you're looking for your partner to have somebody to talk with, that's a fair goal. If you're hoping the preacher can say something that will fix the problem, there's nobody who can do that except your partner himself.

I was not actively religious at the end of my struggles with addiction, and while I have gone a long way to defining my spirituality as part of my recovery, the church has not played an active role in most of my story.

I think an individual's relationship with God is more important than where they sit for an hour on Sundays, although

I absolutely respect your right to disagree. However, as with everything else around recovery, this is largely going to come down to your partner deciding what's right for him.

You should not compromise your religious and spiritual beliefs for him, but he should also not have to compromise his for you. I think it's perfectly fine to suggest he look to God or speak to your pastor, but if he doesn't want to, there really isn't any way to make him.

Does this mean that God is mad at me or doesn't love me?

Tony, the mental health professional:

Absolutely not. I believe this beyond a shadow of a doubt. His heart breaks for you. He weeps for you. You are a Child of God, and as a parent, don't you want the best for your child? I believe, after working with over 1,000 pornography addicts, that this is one of the biggest lies they are telling themselves, that God has given up on them, that He doesn't love them, or that He is mad at them.

I am a huge believer in the evidence-based counseling modality called Acceptance and Commitment Therapy (ACT). Simplified, you can set a goal to put pornography behind you once and for all, and that feels good. Your brain squirts a bit of dopamine, a feel-good chemical, to the reward center of your brain, and for a short time you feel like this time it's going to be different, you're going to exercise, eat right, read scriptures and pray morning and night. Shortly after that initial "rush," ACT teaches that you then can sit back.

I believe that Christ-like love is unconditional love and you know that God will never give up on you. He's always there for you.

I think asking yourself this question either comes from shame you're feeling or from it being put upon you by others. This is wrong because it can lead to more shame and more isolation.

It's understandable that you're asking this question because you're in a pattern of negative thinking right now. Is he angry with you? Does he want to punish you? It's actually quite the opposite.

Josh, the former pornography addict:

Much like you have to understand that your partner's addiction doesn't have anything to do with you, you need to understand that God isn't mad at you and hasn't stopped loving you for a condition another person is struggling with.

Do you think God gets mad at the wife of someone with leukemia or cancer? I can't believe that's the case, even if the person with the health condition did things (like smoking) to bring upon their fate. My God isn't mad at the smoker, much less his girlfriend or wife.

I understand that the practice of looking at pornography is a sin for most believers, but if you want to nit-pick, there is sin throughout all of our lives. I have a hard time believing He is going to pick this one and blame you. That's not the Higher Power I worship.

I think you need to look at this as a test, or a series of tests. The first is whether you stay or not. Maybe God is testing you to see if you'll stay or go. Maybe he's testing your patience. Maybe he's not testing anything that has to do with you, and just like addiction itself, this is all about your partner.

I don't know exactly what God you pray to, but mine doesn't get mad at me and could never not love me.

Can't I just pray this away?

Tony, the mental health professional:

I almost want to be flippant and say, "So how's that worked for you so far?" I find that when I deal with couples, when they ask a version of this question, it's because they don't want to do the hard work involved with getting healthy. They typically aren't doing the work that needs to get done.

I've seen faith-based support groups where people hold their hands out to the sky, saying things like, "God, why have your forsaken me?" when they are in the throes of addiction. It's okay to do that, but I feel like asking, "Why weren't you praying about this a lot earlier?"

I think faith has an important role in recovery, as does praying, but it really comes down to being willing to do the hard work. If you're in a good place spiritually, the hard work may not seem as hard.

Praying for hope, strength and faith can be a great thing for the spiritually-inclined person on their road to recovery.

I think God wants you to do well, but I think God also knows you have to put in the work. I believe that God and Jesus both love you and are not trying to punish you. I know there are some people of different faiths who will say this is a punishment of God, but I disagree.

Josh, the former pornography addict:

Well, there are pockets of the world where religious miracles have been as close to verified as you can get, and of course, there are people who miraculously recover from terminal illnesses. So, I can't say that you can't pray it away, but I look at praying for miracles the way I look at buying lottery tickets to hit the jackpot. The odds are, it's not going to happen.

If praying away an illness worked, there would be no sick people in this world. How many millions of hours have been spent praying for sick children where the prayers seemingly went unanswered? How many millions of people with cancer have died with plenty of prayers behind them?

I think you can pray for guidance and strength, but praying that his addiction—which is a physical disease of the brain—will be miraculously taken away is a recipe for disaster. History tells us that you're not going to be the one-in-a-million who has a miracle happen.

I know that many people have prayed for my recovery and here I am, doing a great job with it. Maybe a gradual improvement is more realistic to pray for, along with the strength for your partner to stick to a recovery plan.

I think that prayer can be a useful tool for many people to get through the recovery process, but I think it can't be the only mode of treatment.

I believe God wants me to stay, but I want to leave. What should I do?

Tony, the mental health professional:

When people are sitting in my office and ask this question, or any variation of it, I sometimes call it, "Playing the Holy Ghost Card." By this I mean, who am I, the therapist, or who is your Pastor, or parent, or friend, to try and trump God when it comes to what is best for you?

It is important at times to reframe the situation. There's been betrayal trauma thrust upon the woman and she feels torn between going and staying. It really is a question of if (assuming the male partner is on board) they are willing to invest the time into changing the dynamics of the relationship and trying to get to a version of the relationship that doesn't have this addiction as part of it.

This question often comes up when an addict is not doing the work, but the spouse is scared to enforce any boundaries, including leaving. He isn't rebuilding trust and she often doesn't know what to do. This is when I inevitably hear, "God has told me to stay."

However, over the last few years, having been through this plenty of times, I have gotten to the point where I can tell them I'm not trying to question God, but I sometimes wonder if they could also be feeling a tremendous amount of fear in moving forward without their spouse. If you have kids, if finances are tight, if you are alone in your town, leaving can feel extremely overwhelming.

Remember, your brain truly believes it is acting in your best interest when it desires the path of least resistance. The brain has evolved into a very sophisticated "stay alive" device, and your brain believes that the best way to accomplish this is by avoiding uncomfortable situations.

So, I do wonder aloud with clients if it may be fear that is leading to the feelings of whether or not to stay, or if the client is confident that it's God directing them to stay or leave. Ultimately, for someone of faith or anyone for that matter, the decision is their decision to make. Many people in difficult situations want someone else to tell them what to do. There's a bit of that type of behavior hardwired into us as children. We wanted our parents to take care of us and make hard decisions, but you have to be the one to make this decision. If you are someone who relies on God to help, then only you can make the decision whether the answer truly is from God or one that may possibly be rooted in fear. I stay away from devolving into a theological debate with a client, but from my chair, I can't imagine a God who wants you to stay in an abusive situation. In general terms, I don't think God wants his children to suffer.

Josh, the former pornography addict:

That's a very difficult question. I would step back and try to look at it from a logical perspective. Why does God want you to stay? Because you're supposed to and made a vow? If you're married, that's the case; if you're not married, leaving is a lot easier, but you may still feel like you're supposed to stay and help him through this. I think that's noble, but you're in for a long, rough road that doesn't have the guarantee of success at the finish line.

If you're worried about your vows, I think talking to your pastor about what they really mean and what they cover is a good conversation to have. I have met Men of God who take the position that the Heavenly Father doesn't want you suffering and others who have said "better or worse" is a black-and-white statement.

Much like most contemporary social topics, I'm sure there are people who could find some part of the Bible that says you should stay and another that says you should go.

I guess it comes down to the question of if serving what you think is the will of God is more important than your personal mental and emotional health.

I don't care if you're the most devout believer or you're the biggest atheist on the planet. I would tell someone to try and fix things, and if they can't, to leave.

If your partner isn't going to take their addiction seriously and do anything about it, how can you be expected to stay in that environment? It's not like he's developed cancer and is opting to skip chemotherapy. There are other aspects of abuse that sometimes come with addiction that you shouldn't have to deal with.

I can only speak for myself, but I think my God wouldn't want me to stay. He wants me to do the most good I can in this world and it starts with taking care of myself. If my partner is going to hinder that, I shouldn't be with my partner.

Will we be forced out of church if people find out about him?

Tony, the mental health professional:

This is a shame-based belief or shame-based fear. It's a "nobody else has problems" kind of fear. If you've heard this from your spouse, that tells me that he is worrying about the judgement, guilt and shame of others. It is these types of thoughts that most likely kept him in the addiction, hiding and isolating from others. It's the "everybody will hate me" type of thinking, or the "I'm unlovable" story that most likely has been on repeat in his brain.

Everyone has their individual struggles, battles and problems. I know that there's this dark little piece that lives in a lot of people that tends to come out when they see others fall. Many people gossip, or judge, simply to make themselves feel better or above someone else. I've had couples in my office who say it makes them feels stronger as a couple when they see another couple's marriage hit the skids. This is when I have to worry about throwing stones at glass houses. None of us are perfect and karma can be rough when it's your turn to somehow fall.

If it does become common knowledge within your church, there may be people who you find heaping judgment on you, but if it's like most churches made of a solid, faith-based community, the majority of members will be there to support you and continue to treat you like brothers and sisters.

Some churches do ask their members to meet with a council of leaders, or elders, who may ultimately decide on membership status within the church. Sometimes these councils do temporarily remove membership status, which can add shame to the betrayer, but ultimately no one is "forced out." This may be part of the betrayer's journey back to their faith community.

Josh, the former pornography addict:

Hopefully not and probably not. You likely will be judged by your fellow churchgoers, and you'll have to ask yourself if it's worth getting looks or if you should find another place to worship where they don't know about your dirty laundry.

I once did a podcast with a woman who talked about how a convicted sex offender who did several years in prison for touching a child asked to join their church. After several meetings of church leaders, they agreed to let the man join, but they had several conditions around limiting his access to children and alerting members of the church.

There was another man who was in a support group (although not a 12 Step group) I attended for a few years after I got out of jail who spoke about his place at his church. He also had a contact offense, and they were very strict with him. I thought too strict, but he was willing to accept their rules and regulations to remain a member.

I have never heard of a church of any religion or domination kicking someone out for being a porn addict, and the irony is, according to many statistics, religious people tend to have higher incidents of porn addiction, or at least they report them at a higher rate.

It's probably safe to assume you won't be kicked out because there are plenty of other porn addicts there. If the church adopted a policy of kicking out people who have sinned, there would be nobody left!

The more I pray, the worse his problem gets. Why?

Tony, the mental health professional:

I believe that this question is more about what you are praying for. Are you praying to fix his problem without any work, or are you praying for strength on the journey of recovery? Are you praying with empathy and compassion regarding your partner? Are you praying to feel Christ's love for you, and your partner, or are you praying that he'll simply pull his head out of his you-know-what? Prayer still requires action. It's like praying for your bills to get paid when you don't have a job. Sure, miracles do occur. If you are a person of faith, no doubt you've heard the stories of someone who just spent their last dollar and then they open the mailbox and find a check from a long-lost relative in just the amount they needed. But I believe there is a big difference between someone who prays for the miracle but doesn't put in any effort on their own versus someone who prays for strength to do the things to put themselves in a position for God to bless them. In the world of betrayal trauma, it may not seem fair for you to have to do recovery work, and often times it's not fair, but as you pray for healing, I believe you will be in a much better place to heal if you're doing your own work. With regard to your partner, I believe sincere prayer will most likely not leave you feeling like his problem and your prayers are correlated.

I believe that prayer is not necessarily about asking for tangible things. It's more about trying to bring your will in alignment with the will of God and being able to accept God's will and trusting that God sees a larger picture, that he knows what is best for you. One definition of prayer that I like says that the object of prayer "is not to change the will of

God but to secure for ourselves and for others blessings that God is already willing to grant but that are made conditional on our asking for them."

One of my daughters approached me when she was in 8th grade and shared that she wanted to start doing gymnastics. My immediate reaction was that she was too old. I questioned her commitment with all of the other school activities she was doing, and admittedly, I worried about the financial burden if this was just an impulsive itch she felt needed to be scratched. After asking her more about why she wanted to try gymnastics, she shared with me that she had always wanted to, that she regretted stopping when she was younger, and that she just wanted to try it one time so she wouldn't have regrets. She went on to be very good at tumbling, which led her to the cheer and stunt squads in high school, and as of the writing of this book, she is currently entertaining scholarship offers based on her cheerleading and stunt work, which all began because of her desire to take gymnastics in 8th grade. I was more than happy to accommodate her wishes once she came to me and made her desires known. I believe prayer can work like that, we need to go to God and ask for the desires of our hearts, be prepared for the answer to be "not right now," and then be willing to put in the effort.

I believe that many blessings require effort on our part, and prayer is a form of work, or effort, that was designed to help us receive blessings from a loving God.

Are you praying for the desires of your heart? Are you willing to put in any effort that God requires? Or are you praying out of anger, or spite, toward your spouse? I believe that prayer can be a very powerful tool in moving forward. Prayer is inward work which leads to outward change.

Josh, the former pornography addict:

As I've already mentioned, I'm not the most spiritual person in the world and I rarely say a prayer, but when I do, if I look at it, all I'm saying is, "This is out of my hands and I hope..." When I was sitting in jail, I came to terms with my spirituality, but what that really consisted of was understanding that I believed something with a larger consciousness than we can imagine is out there.

I think that there are things that we can't explain and may never explain. I think there are concepts that the best we can hope for is to understand that we can't understand. Take how small we are in the universe. You are sitting at an address in a city that is part of country, that is part of a planet, solar system, galaxy and universe. Some scientists believe there are many universes. What if universes are as common as the address in the city you're sitting at right now? What if that is only a speck in how big everything really is? It's hard to fathom.

The more you understand the universe, it doesn't change the universe. Heck, the more you understand the history of Northern Ireland, it doesn't change anything about the political climate. Understanding something better doesn't equal resolution.

Along with understanding that there is something bigger out there (which most people call God but I still just call "The Universe"), I also came to recognize that I had a tremendous amount of faith. Even when things are horrible in my life, I always believe they are going to turn out for the better. I believe at any given time I am where I am supposed to be.

The story of my life wasn't one where I became known as a great magazine publisher or politician. Sure, when I was doing those things they were important to me and I thought I'd be doing them the rest of my life, but the only remnants of them in my life today are a couple boxes of magazines and trophies somewhere in my garage.

Now I believe that pornography addiction education and support is what I'm supposed to be doing with my life. Maybe I'll still be doing this in 2032, or maybe I'll be doing something else. Whatever it is I'm doing, it will be exactly what is supposed to happen.

I think praying is a great activity, especially if it gives you a sense of peace and you feel a connection with something bigger, but what you're hoping will happen may not be what is supposed to happen. It may also take more time than you'd expect, but again, it's all happening for a reason.

There's a great consciousness at work here, and it's never wrong.

Tony Overbay & Joshua Shea

Chapter 6
Addressing His Addiction with Him

Can I force him to get help?

Tony, the mental health professional:

You may be able to force him to get help, or move toward help, but unfortunately he needs to want help. Let me be clear. From my experience, and in my training, he needs help. He did not get caught or confess after simply viewing pornography for the first time. Remember, when it comes to betrayal trauma recovery, or simply trying to decide whether or not you want to stay in the relationship, you need to establish boundaries as the betrayed. If one of your boundaries is that you need to see work being done toward his recovery, in that sense, yes, you can "force" him to get help, but again, it's up to him to embrace and engage in the help.

That said, I do feel like there are a lot of women who simply accept, "Yeah, I'm working on it" from their husbands or boyfriends, but often they aren't seeing the work being done and they aren't hearing about the work he does. It is fair for you to ask about his progress, if he's attending group meetings, and generalities about how his individual therapy sessions are going. Many women tell me within a faith-based recovery that they want to see their husband reading scripture and saying prayers. They want it to be sincere, but they want to know that he cares enough for them to put in the effort.

I've worked with men who have been forced into this situation and sometimes them being coerced into therapy is just the wake-up call they need. For other men, they prefer going to some kind of support group because it stirs a feeling of camaraderie or brotherhood.

Having seen over 1,000 addicts, I can boil it down to two kinds of men who come into my office. There are the ones who were caught, recognize they have a problem and say they'll do whatever it takes to rebuild trust and fix their relationship. I usually think to myself, "Okay, I can work with this," because at least he's getting off on the right foot.

Then there is the small percentage of men who say, "I got caught or I told you what I was doing and now it's in the past and you just need to accept it. I don't want you on my case or telling me what to do. You just have to trust me."

Sometimes an ultimatum or being forced is just what your partner needs, and any chance he gets to reflect on his addiction is better than nothing. If he completely fights it, you have a different set of questions to ask yourself.

Josh, the former pornography addict:

There are ways you can manipulate him to change or even disrupt his typical routine, but on a strict legal basis, there's very little you can do. I've met several people in rehab who had a psychotic episode while on drugs and were held for observation by a hospital for 48 or 72 hours, but the odds are your husband or boyfriend isn't out of his mind, even if he has changed from the person you first fell in love with.

If he's doing something illegal (not necessarily connected to his addiction), you could turn him in and hope that it leads to an awakening, but that's a risky move to make. If he's doing something illegal, you need to talk to a lawyer and/or a close confidante to make sure you're safe and liability free of whatever he's doing.

Finally, there are ultimatums. I have talked with a lot of women who caught their husband and basically said, "If you don't quit, or at least get help, then I'm leaving." In many of their cases it worked, but that was only because they were serious about leaving. If you know that this is not a big enough issue for you to leave over, don't threaten it.

In my case, nobody threatened me because the damage had already been done. I found myself with charges of talking to a teenager online. Immediately thereafter, still months before accepting I had a porn addiction, I told my lawyer of my alcoholism and he strongly suggested I find a program immediately.

It wasn't an ultimatum, but I could read between the lines and see that it could only help my case, even if it didn't help me. That was enough for me to pack my things and head across the country. Thankfully, after a week of being hard-headed, I opened my mind to the idea that I might have a drinking problem. That openness was exercised again and again through my recovery process and it's just part of who I am now.

The one thing I would urge you to do is to talk this over with a professional before you make any grand declarations. He may be like one of those men who immediately agree to whatever you want for fear of what may happen next, or he may be a pain in the neck who not only doesn't think he has a problem, but the problem is so acute that he'd throw away the marriage to not admit it exists. A professional can help with your specific situation and work out possible scenarios.

He admitted he's addicted, what now?

Tony, the mental health professional:

If you're asking this question in the few days after you've either confronted him or he's come clean, there are probably a mix of emotions happening, and it's sometimes difficult to know which ones to trust and act on and which others are just fleeting for the moment or perhaps are reinforcing negative thinking or behaviors.

I've seen women wake-up the morning after a late-night admission feeling closer to their partner than they ever had before because they have never felt that emotionally close and they see the conversation revealing a deeper conversation than they knew was there. The odds are he also promised never to look at pornography again.

I've also seen men wake-up the next morning with the attitude of, "I'm glad I told you this and I feel like it's not going to be a problem anymore because I opened up and I feel so relieved. I think we're good on the porn."

He's running through the promise that he's done with it. This is not the first time he's made this promise, but it may be the first time he's made it to you. Making those kinds of promises hasn't worked before, and it's likely not going to work just because he made it to you. Admitting you are an addict is a great first start, but now it's time to get to work.

I had a client not too long ago who was nine months clean and sober from pornography. He didn't touch the stuff, but he also wasn't doing the work. He was scared by his partner into sobriety, but that can only last so long. He had calendar-based success, but not a change of heart. He hadn't changed his relationship with intimacy, with sexuality.

I would bring up the fact he wasn't embracing recovery and he'd just say, "I'm good. I'm good." Around month 10, he wasn't good anymore. It's important to also note that there is a likelihood that after a couple of days, those warm-fuzzy feelings you have are going to wear off and you may swing toward the other end of the spectrum and think, "Holy cow! Has my whole marriage been a lie?" Unfortunately, this is part of the betrayal trauma. It is perfectly fine to have these mood swings. It is part of the process.

After this admission, the next best step is to get a professional involved as soon as possible. It won't guarantee success, but it is somebody who has experience in the field and there are some very solid, evidence-based steps to take throughout the betrayal trauma journey that a professional can help with.

Josh, the former pornography addict:

That's a huge, huge thing. Of course, just saying you have an addiction doesn't actually change anything. I've been told by 100% of the people who have heard me that I'm a terrible singer, but that has never stopped me from grabbing a microphone at karaoke. Unless the behavior changes, all you have is a situation everybody agrees with.

For me, the next move was rehab, because as I mentioned in the last question, I was urged to make a grand gesture to the judge in my case. My motivation was to stay out of jail, or lessen any sentence I'd eventually receive. What are his motivations?

If he is at his best in a group setting, you may urge him to contact the local Sex Addicts Anonymous Group. I attended these meetings while in rehab and for a while once I returned home before I felt they were no longer helping. If he likes one-on-one, have him talk to a therapist. Personally, I wouldn't want my wife in the room when I was talking about this stuff for the first time, so if you do want to do marriage counseling, I wouldn't make it the centerpiece.

If he's admitted he's addicted, let him decide the next steps. They may not be the ones that lead to recovery, but he needs to be the one driving his recovery, not you. Whatever modality of treatment he wants to try, encourage him and support him, even if it's not your first choice.

Remember that this is not like a broken rib. It won't just heal in a few months on its own. You're in for a recovery journey that, if successful, will likely be intense at first, but always be present. My porn addiction is like my alcoholism in that it will always need to be monitored. The further I get from actively being an addict, the easier it gets, but I will never reach a day when I say I am cured.

Does he need to go to inpatient rehab?

Tony, the mental health professional:

I do not claim to be the final say in questions like this. I would definitely recommend that you are working directly with a professional who has significant experience working with men who turn to compulsive sexual behaviors to cope with, or numb out of, life. I have read books and stories about men who have only discovered how bad their addiction was by going to in-patient rehab facilities. My co-author on this book will have a lot to say on this subject. I can only speak to my own experience in working with over 1,000 men who have come to see me specifically for pornography addiction and compulsive sexual behavior.

In my experience, I have worked with roughly a dozen men who have been to inpatient rehab facilities. In all but two of these experiences, these men have attended in order to show their spouses that they were serious about their recovery. In a couple of these situations, the financial impact on the family from the month away from work, as well as the cost of rehab, has been serious and the family struggled to overcome it. I only mention this because if your reason behind insisting that he enter inpatient rehab is, again, that you want him to hurt like you are hurting, then I would talk this over with a mental health professional. If you and your spouse together believe that his addiction seems completely out of his control, then I would suggest thinking long and hard about this decision with someone trained in sexual addiction and compulsive sexual behavior.

In my practice, I have seen three types of men come back from inpatient rehab:

The first had a very positive experience and they think, "I've got this." They had a worthwhile experience, did the work there and understand that regular therapy needs to be part of their relapse prevention plan. The inpatient rehab was truly the wake-up call that they needed, the break, the reset. They needed time away from their triggering environments in order to truly see how deeply they were involved in the addiction. These men come back home appreciative of their new awareness of how they got to where they are now. They are buying into the concepts of therapy in general and self-discovery, and they are owning their own part in the addiction. These people will typically continue to attend therapy and recognize that these changes are good for them, not just good for them because they may be able to save their families, but good for them because they deserve to live a life free of turning toward instant gratification to cope with stressors. Inpatient rehab truly was the catalyst to get things moving in positive directions in his life.

The second kind of guy comes out of rehab and says, "I'm cured!" They may have had a similar experience to the first guy, but they believe that dozens of hours of therapy over a month at an inpatient facility is equal to dozens of hours of therapy over a year in my office. These are often the guys who get thrown a bit when life starts to come back and challenge them. They feel like they're completely different and expect the world to be as well. They often feel that they are "done" when they get home. Needless to say, I often see these men remain sober for months, sometimes even years, but ultimately, without staying on the work, they tend to relapse.

Then there are the people who went and "painted-by-the-numbers," so to speak, meaning they attended the meetings, did the group art projects, "participated," but largely ignored everything they worked on while they were there. They come back to the same negative relationships and the same job they don't like. They "did their time" and they aren't happy about it, but they made it through, so basically everybody needs to "back off" and let them try and get back to work. If you're not reading this with sarcasm, please go back, restart this paragraph and do so. It's hard to tell if they went into it with a bad attitude or if they just faked their way through it.

Josh, the former pornography addict:

If he wants to go, then I would encourage him. If he doesn't want to go, it probably is worth a conversation with a professional so they can weigh-in to decide which way to take things.

I probably urge people to go to inpatient rehab quicker than most, but that's because my two stints, first for alcohol and a year later for porn, were the most transformative experiences of my life. Both times I walked into the facility as one person and walked out somebody else.

It's easy to make excuses why he shouldn't go. He has a job, he helps with the kids, and he's got other responsibilities. I would counter that needing a break to take care of one's health is just as important as all of those things.

My wife ran the house when I did my 10-week and 7-week stints at inpatient rehab. Thankfully, we were in a financial position where that was possible, but even if we didn't have savings, I would have found a way. I would have asked for help from family and friends. People don't want to ask, but others generally like to help people who are helping themselves.

I've encountered so many people who make excuses why they can't go to rehab, and while they are almost always valid, I also bring up the point that my wife ran the household for six months while I served my jail sentence. In that case, I did have to ask my parents for help, and it wasn't a surprise when they were there for us.

With jail, I didn't have a choice. What would happen if your partner was caught for drunk driving and sentenced to 30 days? Would your world implode? Probably not. You'd figure it out and you'd get through it. My wife is proof of that.

I actually think the time that I was away was like a rehab for my family. They needed time away from my energy and my illness. They needed to reconnect instead of hovering around me like satellites. I actually made the comment to my wife that they all seemed to be far more functional and healthy when I wasn't there during that period.

I know people who have had successful recovery having never stepped foot into rehab, and I know plenty of people who have never been able to get into a recovery groove despite having gone to rehab five or six times.

I truly believe I would not have had the strength to maintain recovery as well as I did had I not gone to rehab and begun the process of understanding how I became the person I did. Maybe I would have reached the same place over a longer time period with just one-on-ones and group therapy at home, but I know just how much inpatient rehab did for me.

Should we go to couple's counseling?

Tony, the mental health professional:

As a couple's therapist this is a difficult one. My first answer wants to be YES you need to figure out where the wedges formed in the relationship, but I recognize now, after years of betrayal trauma training and extensive couples therapy training, that if a couple is not in a position to BOTH work on themselves and the relationship, then sitting down for couples counseling can actually be contra-indictated, meaning it can do additional damage.

Imagine being in a session with a spouse who just discovered that her husband has been lying about a pornography addiction for 20 years of marriage and that his addiction gradually led him to not only pull away from the family, due to his own shame, but into a relationship with someone who he now says "gets him." This is a scenario that I see all too often when couples first come into counseling when they have presented as simply needing "couple's therapy" to improve communication. In reality, there was significant betrayal trauma discovered in the relationship.

So, my first recommendation is to have the betrayed seek counseling with someone who is trained in working with betrayal trauma, someone who has training in working with compulsive sexual behaviors. I also recommend that the betrayer seek counseling immediately with someone who is equally trained. If your individual therapists are not part of a group of therapists who treat these issues specifically, I would highly recommend having each of you sign a release so that your therapists can share information, but again, your therapists must be trained in this area! The goal of the release is not to share information to use against the partner in their own therapy, but more to assess where the individuals are in their own therapy to begin talk of possible couple's therapy.

Josh, the former pornography addict:

I attended couples counseling a long time ago in two different chunks. First was early in my marriage when we just hit some kind of funk, or at least I did. I think I just needed to shake it off and don't recall much good coming from that therapist.

The second therapist we saw was better. He helped us to get at our core issues of the time, which on my end was how my wife spent money and on her end was how much I helped around the house. Not exactly exotic problems, but they were holding us back.

I have to admit, we didn't go through the entire therapy cycle or reach a point where the therapist told us that we had made progress and could cut down on visits. After five or six sessions, we agreed together to quit.

I think those sessions helped, but I also think that we were just struggling with communication more than anything else. Once we got that back on track, there wasn't much of a reason to continue forward in our opinions.

Of course, being who I was at the time, in the ongoing phase of porn addiction—yet still years away from recognizing I actually had an addiction—I wasn't about to mention during the therapy that I was indulging in pornography three-to-five nights a week, many times choosing it over actual sexual contact.

You probably feel a giant sense of betrayal, and he's likely feeling a cadre of emotions as well. If he offers to go to couple's counseling, I'd say go for it. If he is hesitant, accept his hesitancy and see a counselor on your own.

A couple's counselor is only going to be as good as your husband or boyfriend is honest. Your significant other may need to talk about this to somebody one-on-one before he feels comfortable discussing it in front you.

I'd also urge you to think about this. You're going to hear a lot of things that you may not be ready to hear yet. You may hear things you're not at the place to believe and process.

Most couple's counselors are smart enough to hold individual sessions with each member of the couple prior to bringing them together. If you go first, express your concerns about the process. You don't want to send your partner running.

I think almost all counseling is good, but I think you need to want to be there and be an active member. If he sits there like a bump on a log refusing to say anything, that's not helping the situation.

My wife and I never did couple's counseling as part of my recovery, and I don't think we suffered for it. We both went to individual therapists, and my wife and kids went to my therapist for a few family sessions while I was in jail. It sounded like it went well and was good to have someone who knew so much of my history leading my family through a difficult time.

I think couple's counseling is another tool or modality for people to consider. It will be the absolute answer that solves all of the problems for some, and for others it will be a waste of money. There's nothing wrong with finding out if it's one of those two or somewhere in the middle.

He says he wants help, but I think he just wants to stay together. What do I do?

Tony, the mental health professional:

It's normal that you're assuming the worst. You're probably trying to figure out what else has been a lie in your marriage, or at least wondering if he's manipulated you into believing other things aren't true.

At this fragile time in your marriage, and in the very beginning stages of what will hopefully be a successful recovery, it's hard to know the way things should unfold vs. the way things will unfold.

From my experience, saying he needs help is a good place to start from, even if you're suspect of the intention. You're going to be suspect of every intention for a while, perhaps even a long while.

It's also okay to let him know that you're not sure he's telling you he wants help for his own good and the sake of your relationship, or if he's just saying it because he's scared of things changing.

This is one of those situations where I urge having a third-party professional available when some of these conversations are happening. I'll have guys who come in for their third or fourth appointment with their wife saying things like, "I've been good for two or three weeks now and she's still not calming down. I just want her to relax. I want her to go back to the old way things were."

When I hear something like that, I know that the wife's first instinct that husband wasn't really looking for help for the right reasons is correct.

There are various avenues I can take the couple down if that is the case, but I think it's important to initially give him the benefit of the doubt while you start to deal with your own betrayal trauma recovery.

Josh, the former pornography addict:

As both Tony and I mention elsewhere in this book, there are a percentage of men who, when confronted about their addiction, are suddenly relieved and ready to seek help. The one person who they didn't want to find out—you—did, and now they can do something about it. They want to get healthy and they want to be part of a solid team.

Then there are the guys who say they want to get help, but who seem to not want to upset the apple cart. "Okay, you found out, but I like our life and I'll quit because I like our life." These are the guys who will attempt to quit, and may even be successful for a while.

I saw a lot of these men as newcomers at Sex Addicts Anonymous meetings. They'd show up for a month or two and then disappear. I didn't follow-up with any of them, but I had a feeling that they heard stories much worse than theirs, evaluated their situation, and came to the conclusion that their biggest fault was that they got caught.

If he's not looking to truly, actually work on his problem, and he's just more concerned with maintaining the status quo, you're going to find yourself exactly where you are right now at some point in the near future.

He's really just gaslighting you in a completely different way. Instead of denying there's any problem, he's going to admit there's a problem and talk about how well he is taking care of it. Now that his secret is out and confirmed, he can't try to act like it's not happening. It makes more sense to him to say he has a problem and say he's taking care of it.

What most addicts are looking for, and I know I was for years, is the path of least resistance. I can't count the number of times that I have told people my motto for life was, "Don't ask permission, just say you're sorry after the fact." It was easier for me to shrug and act charming having done the wrong thing than to do the right thing in the first place. This is probably the head-space your partner is in right now.

He could be gaslighting his therapist, if he's even showing up for the sessions. He could be just looking at the clock at his Sex Addicts Anonymous meetings, discounting what the others are saying. He could also be sitting in an Arby's parking lot enjoying curly fries and playing on his phone while you think he's at the meeting.

This goes back to the fact that you may need to create boundaries, issue ultimatums and enforce penalties for not respecting your boundaries or ignoring your ultimatums.

If your partner shows no interest in truly getting better, you may have to be the conduit for change.

Does counseling or inpatient rehab actually work?

Tony, the mental health professional:

In general, the answer is yes, but the outcome falls on his shoulders. If he is earnest in wanting to recover, it's possible. I'll sit down with men who have tried to quit on their own, but to no avail. When left to their own devices, they often can't battle the beast of addiction.

It really takes someone who is willing to say, "I have a problem and I want to solve it. Who I am is not the person I want to be." That's somebody who is starting off on the right foot and seems like they're willing to put the work in.

Wanting to put the work in on your own is a noble idea, but I see that fail so much more than I see it succeed. In this world where we Google away all of our problems, it's almost too much to face the world of information out there.

Those keyboard warriors seem to think that the answer is just white-knuckling it, but kicking an addiction like pornography is not like trying to stop smoking. If you're white-knuckling it and going cold turkey without professional help, you're not getting to the core issues of the addiction. You can deal with the symptoms, but that's not going to touch upon what really needs to be addressed.

Josh, the former pornography addict:

Yes. Counseling and rehab saved my life, and I urge anybody reading this to get yourself a therapist, no matter how healthy you think you are. When the spotlight is turned on you and you're free to babble for 42 minutes about nothing in particular, it's sometimes amazing what comes out of your mouth at minute 43. As it turns out, you weren't babbling. You were making connections and eventually made a connection you hadn't considered before. I call these the "A-ha! Moments," and they are some of the most eye-opening, amazing moments in therapy.

Like every other form of help, the person seeking the help actually needs to want it. There is no form of therapy that will help somebody 100% of the time if they are fighting it.

I started going to therapists when I was about 20 years old, following the death of one of my best friends. I got a few tools for dealing with the immediate problem, but then I was in-and-out of therapy for the next 15 years. I was eventually diagnosed bipolar around 25 and thought that might mean the end of therapy, but it was still something I needed.

The problem was, I was only 90% honest with my therapist. I cut out the most negative details of my life and can now also see that I had repressed many memories that never surfaced because the people I saw didn't have the schooling to identify I was carrying those memories.

It wasn't until rehab, when I was in therapy every day, that I made the connection that I really had to do the hard work. I had to do the digging, I had to do the analysis, and I had to make the changes. For 15 years, I was waiting for a therapist to reveal the silver-bullet that would explain my existence.

That magical statement doesn't exist, and I think about the time I wasted in therapy waiting to hear it. I believed one day I'd hear, "Because you are X, you must Y and you will be happy." I thought it would be as simple as that.

Therapy is about examining issues in your life, looking at different ways of addressing those issues and figuring out which is the best. It's about sharing what's happening with your life, and in the process of sharing, understanding what takes priority.

I liken therapy to the process of editing a book. What you're reading right now is the shortest version of this book that ever existed. There were many things that either Tony or I wrote that we decided were unimportant to the theme of the book. Then, of course, there are editors and publishers who made their own cuts.

In the first book I wrote, I had over 200,000 words in the first draft. The final published book is about 85,000 words. The process of cutting was eye-opening, because it forced me to make decisions on what was important, what I really wanted to say and what the message of the book was. I think therapy is a lot like that. You can't tell a therapist everything that has happened to you, even with years of weekly two-hour sessions. You're forced to self-edit, and just that process of self-editing can be powerful if you take a hard look at it.

I was open to the experiences of inpatient rehab and remain open to the experience of therapy. I can't imagine a life where it is not a vital part of my week. Some sessions are just chit-chat and some sessions feel like being dragged through a swamp. The swamp sessions are the most important.

I can't imagine that I would ever have been able to say I have a healthy life—which I now actually have—without having been to rehab and without making therapy an ongoing priority.

He doesn't want to go to therapy. Should I still go?

Tony, the mental health professional:

Absolutely. You're going to need tools to understand what is happening with addiction and how to deal with it. You're also going to want someone to help you with the betrayal trauma recovery aspects and simply be there to navigate you through whatever is next.

The first time I sit down with a woman going through this, there's often a level of shame and embarrassment about having to see somebody and doing it without her husband. I explain to them they're doing the best thing because right now is a horrible time to be left alone to deal with this in her head.

The one thing I do want to touch upon is to urge you to make sure you're going to a therapist that has experience with addiction and knows their stuff with betrayal trauma. I had a woman come to me once who shared that the first therapist she saw heard her story and asked if perhaps she just wasn't having enough sex with her husband.

A lot of times you'll get a generalist who just doesn't have the experience you need in this situation. I feel like after seeing 1,000 clients, I have enough reps under my belt that I know what to say and what not to say, and if you're just the third client who has a husband with a porn addiction, you may not get the proper attention you need.

I also feel that while a spiritual leader can certainly help counsel you, there are some who go with shame-based solutions and others who take a more positive route. I'm all about being positive, so if you think your priest, reverend, rabbi or whatever will support you, consider talking to them. If they seem like they may be the other way, hold off talking to them about it. I've seen situations where a spiritual leader says the wrong thing and it sets a person back.

Josh, the former pornography addict:

I don't think it will come as any shock to you that I answer this with a resounding, "Yes!"

I believe that even though I wasn't 100% honest with my therapists through my 20s and early 30s, they were still instrumental in helping me get through some of the challenges I faced that had nothing to do with my addictions. There is something powerful about somebody who is there to advocate for you, is rooting for you, but isn't emotionally involved, nor playing an active role in your everyday real life.

The relationship between a therapist and patient is unique and unlike any other. I think most people fear going to a therapist because they think it will be a complete bearing of their deepest secrets, and simply by the act of seeing a therapist, it must mean there is something wrong.

I wish that I could go back to the beginning when I was 20 years old and the therapist inevitably asked me if there was any sexual dysfunction. I could say, "I have been renting porno movies or buying *Playboy* every month since I was 14 years old." I don't know what I thought the blowback would be. They weren't going to kick me out of their office.

But, like so many guys who believed porn was something to be ashamed of and that I was just walking around with this invisible black cloud of perversion over my head, I kept quiet when it came to the pornography. I didn't talk about any of my sexual hang-ups, either. I just said everything was fine and complained about work or my parents.

Would I have ended up behind bars if I had been honest with my therapist in my 20s? Honestly, I don't think so. Part of the reason my addiction festered into a nasty wound was because I never had the salve of a professional's ear. That's on me, not them.

A therapist is a great sounding board, and somebody who isn't going to take it personally when you get mad or start crying or blurting things that you can't believe are coming out of your mouth because you've tried to suppress them for so long. A therapist is going to know the next thing to say to keep things moving in the right direction.

I will mention that, not counting the pair of couple's counselors that my wife and I saw, I've seen five therapists, but I say I've only had two. I probably saw the other three a combined eight times.

If you're not clicking with a therapist, find someone else. In your case, it would help if you could talk to someone who has experience working with relationships and hopefully has some experience in dealing with addiction, even if it is drugs and alcohol. Your personalities must mesh, and there needs to be the opportunity for a level of trust to develop. You're wasting your time if you don't have a bond, or at least I was.

Ironically, the therapist I have now, who has seen me through all of my recovery, is the first woman I've seen. I never would have guessed it, but it isn't an older man who I clicked with, but a woman only a couple years older than me.

You're going to learn a lot about yourself in therapy you never otherwise would have. I wholeheartedly endorse therapy for anyone with a pulse.

Chapter 7
Heading into Recovery

Should I ask to see his online history from now on or put filters on his computer and phone?

Tony, the mental health professional:

If that is a boundary you want to create while he works on his addiction, I think it's a perfectly reasonable thing to ask him to do. However, I do want to make you aware that most addicts have higher-than-average computer skills, and if he doesn't know how to get around filters and he truly is not in a place to work on his addiction, he may try and pick up this skill.

However, even if he is able to work his way around the security, expressing this desire is an extra step in him getting to the pornography. Perhaps that little filler of time is just enough space to allow him to use his tools of recovery and stop before acting out as he's done previously.

Many men who sit down with me who are completely open about their addiction will say they are willing to cooperate with their partner in any way and their partner can view their internet history, look at the texts on their phones, track their car, or whatever else they want to do. I had a guy who offered to wear a webcam 24/7 so his wife could always see what he was up to at any given moment, because he wanted to be transparent. Sometimes I refer to this guy as a guy who "gets it."

These are the men who are often initially glad they got caught. They know they're about to embark on a painful journey, but they also know they can now get the help they need to overcome their addiction.

If there's hard pushback that you're violating his trust or that he doesn't need to be policed, that should cause some red flags, because it's my experience that those reactions are typically from somebody who doesn't plan on staying in recovery (if they enter at all) or who doesn't want to analyze what has caused them to get to this point.

If he's not willing to show you his computer history, texts or anything else you request, he's still not at the point where he's willing to really just be completely honest and open about his addiction.

The one warning I'll give is that the guy who does allow full and open access still may be able to access pornography a number of other ways. You're simply never going to be able to keep it away from him 100%, but setting up certain parameters is not a bad thing.

Josh, the former pornography addict:

One of the methods in early recovery that many people feel is helpful is to have some sort of accountability partner. I don't think the wife should fill this role, but I don't think it's inappropriate to ask to see his online history.

I see this as an exercise that will make you feel better than him. I probably had access to eight devices in my house and another handful at work, but I only used one laptop to look at porn. Had my wife wanted to lock everything down, it would have been a lot of wasted effort. If the police hadn't come and she discovered my use and wanted to put filters on my computer or view my history, I would have told her to go for it.

I would have told myself that she couldn't put filters on the computers at work. In the worst-case scenario, I could easily take the company credit card and go buy myself another phone or laptop if I wanted, since I ran the place.

The more likely scenario would have been that I just got around the filters. I know they're supposed to be foolproof, but I can't tell you how many addicts—both men and women—have told me that filters on computers are security blankets for the partner. They don't actually stop the addict.

I think this is basically the same answer when people ask me if they should put filters on their computers for their kids. Perhaps in a best-case scenario, you lock down one computer. How many millions does that leave out there?

There are corner stores, adult book stores, strip clubs, the list goes on and on, where he can get his addiction fed. Realistically, you can never stop him from accessing pornography.

So why do I think it's not a horrible idea? Because it gives him a moment of pause. If it takes him 10 extra seconds to get around the filters on the computer, that's 10 seconds he has to think about what he's about to do. If your following-up forces him to buy a magazine at the corner store, he has a few minutes to reflect.

You can't stop him, but you can throw a few roadblocks in his way. I believe that's better than nothing.

Will I ever be able to trust him again?

Tony, the mental health professional:

Probably, but it's going to take work on both sides, and one of the most difficult things to remember is that he has to want to do the work necessary to help you feel like you can trust him again. I've worked with over 1,000 men and probably half of that number of couples who have gone through this difficult period of time, and the overwhelming majority go on to have a relationship that they never knew they could have, one full of communication and honesty, which eventually rebuilds trust. This is assuming that the guy is ready to work on the issue, and willing to do whatever it takes to repair the relationship.

In order to get there, I strongly urge the woman to seek her own help and to explore her relationship with trust and learn how to deal with betrayal trauma. Unfortunately, trust can be part of larger "attachment wounds," or struggles to trust people throughout their lives, which can make this process extremely difficult. The one person that they were hoping to finally trust with everything they had, their spouse, had now become another person who has betrayed their trust.

I had a couple who I had been seeing for about a year. The husband made his phone, email, calendar, you name it, open to his wife. He was regularly going to his support groups and was meeting with an individual therapist. By all counts, he was doing the hard recovery work necessary.

His wife had her own therapist to cope with betrayal recovery work, and while I wasn't privy to those discussions, she really seemed to hit a wall when it came to trust.

The husband started to get frustrated because he felt that he had done everything that he had been asked to do and that he knew to do in his recovery, but he was still being subjected to line after line of questioning, sometimes for hours. He felt like there were only so many times he could provide an answer to, "How could you have done this to me?"

The bottom line is that things will never be the same. But if he's doing all of the work and everything asked of him, you've got to be willing to shift a little and go a little deeper with those thoughts of betrayal trauma, because they may not just be about him.

I struggle asking anything of the wife who has been betrayed early on. Her world has been turned upside down with the disclosure. If she wasn't feeling emotional instability throughout the day, even sometimes throughout the hour, I would question whether or not she was truly dealing with her emotions. But if he is truly being open, being honest, and trying to do the work necessary, the work asked of him, I do begin to ask the wife to perhaps take a deeper look at why she is struggling so hard to move forward—not to move on, not to forgive and forget, but to move forward.

I love Acceptance and Commitment Therapy (ACT) as a therapy model for individuals. In simplistic terms, when we decide we're going to do something that generally lines up with our individual values, the brain will shoot a bit of dopamine to the reward center. So, if he's truly trying to do the work asked, the wife may say, "Okay, I think our relationship is going well. I think we're going to make this work!" There goes that shot of dopamine.

But remember, your brain's job is to try and protect you. So as soon as that dopamine shot occurs, the brain goes into "reason giving" mode, meaning it will now quickly give you all of the reasons why the relationship is not going to work. "What if he does it again? What if my friends are disappointed that I let him back in? What if people in our church congregation find out?"

In ACT, we often say that the brain is trying to "hook" you to one of these stories that the brain is telling you. If your brain can hook you to a story, get you to fuse to that story, then you don't have to do the difficult work of letting him back in and continuing to trust him despite the betrayal. Your brain wants the path of least resistance, and right now that would be to not trust him again.

I often ask women to truly look at the stories the brain is trying to get them to fuse to. Are those stories true or false? In ACT that is not the debate, he may do it again, people will probably find out, your friends will have a variety of opinions, but what we're truly trying to determine is whether or not those stories are productive or workable thoughts toward the goal of getting back together or the goal of giving the relationship a true effort of reconciliation.

If you're not familiar with ACT, I would highly recommend the book *The Confidence Gap*, by Russ Harris. *The Confidence Gap* covers the basics of Acceptance and Commitment Therapy in a very easy-to-read format that teaches you more about forming true values-based goals and how to detatch from those unproductive thoughts.

Josh, the former pornography addict:

That's hard to say because I don't know you and I don't know him. I think that my wife is back to trusting me as much as she can, and honestly, as much as she should.

Perhaps this is a jaded view, but I trust her 99%. I think she trusts me 94%, and I think those are very appropriate numbers considering our history.

When you trust somebody 100% it means they are never going to surprise you. It means that they will never act outside of your expectations and there will never be fault in anything they do. Trusting somebody completely is dangerous and it is how people get emotionally crippled, because while you trust unconditionally, the other person may not be able to live up to that lofty standard you've set.

I'd suggest looking back over the rest of your life. Have there been times when somebody has let you down, disappointed you, lied or fully betrayed you? What is your relationship like with that person now?

If you've never been able to mend fences, it's not to say that it's impossible here, but history is generally a good guide of how we're going to act. If it takes you a while, but you eventually forgive and forget, there's a decent chance that you'll be able to trust him in the future.

I think that not trusting him fully in the short-term is actually the smart thing to do. This is a man who, while perhaps dealing with a mental illness, has also been fully engaged in deceit against you. Even if the only thing he did was lie about his pornography use/addiction, that's still one more than a partner should lie about.

I'm not a needle in a haystack as far as success stories go. I have met dozens of couples who have decided to stay together and get things back on the right track. Sure, there are some who simply can't make it through the wreckage of his addiction, but there are a lot who do.

I will say, however, if you think that there is no way that you'll ever be able to forgive him and trust him again, or if you have given it a shot and it's not working, don't give up hope just yet. See if he's open to getting professional help with you. If you have tried professional help and that's not working, you may just sadly be in the percentage of people who let this tear them apart.

I appreciate that to earn the last few percentage points and reach 99% I'm going to have to prove myself to my wife over a series of years. I think that's the way it should be. I deceived her for so long, regaining trust shouldn't be a sprint. It should be a marathon. Eventually, I will get there, but I'm only running because I know I can reach the goal.

Is it okay for him to watch movies with nudity from now on?

Tony, the mental health professional:

This is a choice that the two of you will have to make, again, because everyone has their own boundaries and beliefs around nudity in movies, just like people have differing opinions on violence, foul language and other controversial subjects. First, is he capable of watching a movie with that type of content, and second, how does that affect you? In a securely attached relationship, you should both be able to express your true feelings on the matter. If nudity is extremely triggering for you and he simply says that he wants to watch a movie with nudity, then I would hope that, in order to secure the connection between you, he would understand that watching a movie is not as important as his relationship with you.

If you are against him seeing these movies, that's a perfectly acceptable boundary. There are thousands of good movies to watch, but if he has to choose one that has nudity and he knows it makes you upset, it makes me wonder if he's serious about recovery and your relationship. He's saying that seeing something flash across a screen is more important than the betrayal trauma trigger that may go off in your head.

In all truth, I'd advise him to stay away from those movies because you never know what a trigger is going to be. I've worked with enough addicts to know he could be watching an innocuous movie where there are two seconds of breasts, or he could see an Instagram of a woman in a bikini, and suddenly he's triggered for the first time in months.

I feel like this is the kind of question where, if you have to ask, the answer is no. There are so many other options of things you can do together or movies you can watch that there shouldn't be a need to worry about nudity in what you're viewing.

Josh, the former pornography addict:

Well, that all depends on what his triggers were and how he handles them. I grew up in an age where if you didn't subscribe to HBO, Cinemax or The Playboy Channel, they still came to the house in "scrambled" formats. The audio was clear as day and the picture was usually messed up, but not always.

One of our sports channels, every night at 10 p.m., would flip to scrambled Playboy Channel, then flip back at 6 a.m. One morning I was up early, I happened upon the scrambled channel. All of a sudden, it unscrambled. I looked at the clock. It was 5:55 a.m.

I guess to make sure the other channel was unscrambled at the right time, the cable company cleared the signal early. Armed with this knowledge, I programmed my VCR to record The Playboy Channel from 5:55 a.m. to 6 a.m. every morning for the next month. By the end of the month, I was sitting on almost three hours of porn.

As my story indicates, television and movies were a huge source for my pornography. Being in central Maine, we had a few French-language channels direct from Quebec, Canada. One of them was very liberal with foreign independent film nudity. My middle and high school years were spent flipping back and forth between *Saturday Night Live* and whatever TV5Monde was airing.

I was actually surprised that not very long into recovery, I was able to see incidental nudity in a movie or TV show and not get excited. I felt no rush, nor did it trigger me to run and seek out a celebrity nudity website, which were among my favorites in my early 20s.

The only explanation I have for not feeling anything, and still not really caring to this day, is that I fried my dopamine receptors off of TV and movies a long time ago. When I was in my 20s, I would sit through absolute garbage for an hour if there was a promise of nudity at minute 61. By the time the police intervened when I was 37, I hadn't looked at anything made by a legitimate TV or movie studio in years to meet my pornography needs.

It may be okay for him to watch nudity on TV or in movies, but it may also be the thing that sets him back. If he's open to talking to you, ask him what his triggers are and how you can make life easier for him at home. If that means getting rid of cable, then get rid of cable.

If he's uncomfortable talking about his triggers, use your head and try to observe how he reacts if you're watching a program and there is nudity. His non-verbal reaction probably will provide the answer you're looking for.

Should I just get a divorce, or break up with him, and move on?

Tony, the mental health professional:

This is an incredibly difficult time, so I recommend holding off on making decisions like this until you can get some solid ground under your feet. You may feel like you immediately need space from him in order to process the wave emotions that you are feeling and that are sure to come, but immediately saying that you want a divorce may be somewhat reactionary.

While it's important to council with friends, family and loved ones, just understand that, again, nobody understands all of the individual experiences that have brought you to this point in your life, so it wouldn't be appropriate to expect that anyone can make this decision for you. It's normal, and it can be a good idea, to seek the counsel of trusted friends and family, but avoid those who are going to tell you what you "should" do. I often say in my practice, and on my podcasts, "nobody likes to be should on!"

Obviously, if there are children involved in the relationship, it can become a more complicated question to ask yourself, but I find if women take a few days, they usually come around to the place that they say, "If he's willing to do the work, I'm willing to do the work. This is the man I married, or this is the man I'm planning to marry."

If you're still convinced, after giving some time for the dust to settle, to see what he is willing to do to repair the relationship—barring that there is no safety issue for you—I still urge you to wait. Pick out a block of time, be it 90 days or six months, where you'll just put the idea of leaving or divorce off to the side. That doesn't mean that you have to sleep in the same bed, the same room or even the same house; I'm simply saying to make sure you're in a good place emotionally before making such a large decision.

What you're looking for is if there's a chance at recovery. If divorce or leaving is always at the front of your mind, with the way that brain works, anytime there is discomfort or a trigger, the immediate response in the neuropathways will be that you should leave.

During that block of time, don't ruminate on leaving. I've seen situations where he is doing all the work, but the wife or girlfriend won't let go of the question of if she should leave. Don't just sit there with these thoughts, because they can be toxic.

I feel like the overwhelming majority of people I work with stay in the marriage when the husband does the work because they rediscover what led them to want to get married. It's not just like one day you bumped into your husband

and decided then and there to get married. You developed deep feelings over time that are probably still there. If they weren't, this situation wouldn't feel so bad.

Between doing the hard work to fix things and leaving, I understand that leaving can seem like the easy thing to do... that's because it is. There is a long, uphill climb ahead for both of you. There will be times where you don't trust him, where you wonder if he's relapsed and you wonder if he's really doing the work. It's a daunting task to look at what's ahead, but that's why I urge people to break it into small pieces and work on a piece at a time.

Josh, the former pornography addict:

Ninety percent of me says no. If there's no way that you can ever get through this, or if he has no plan on changing and you can't live with that decision, then maybe it is time to call it quits before things get too heated and stressful.

I'm not there to judge your position, and while I know my wife took a fair amount of flack from people who couldn't understand why she would stay with me, I never felt that my marriage was in danger. That was a huge, huge help to my recovery.

When I was at both rehabs working on getting the tools to be a healthier person, I never had to fear that a call home would result in the horrible news that she was walking away. When I was in jail for six months, I never feared when I saw our return address on a letter from home.

I saw people in rehab, and especially jail, who were not lucky enough to have that sense of a secure relationship that I did. It added another layer to everything they were struggling with. Some shared their stories and some preferred to keep the domestic strife to themselves, but one thing was universal, regardless of time or place: These guys were having a harder time dealing with whatever problem brought them to rehab or jail than they would have without the additional stress.

On family visiting day at either rehab, you could almost set your watch by the arguments that would break out. It meant that an hour had elapsed. When half the patients were crying, it meant that the three hours were up and they were reduced to ravaged chunks of themselves.

In jail, nobody ever let down their guard enough to be seen crying, but the visiting room could get downright hostile. Once returned to the pod, that inmate was usually a seething, boiling kettle for the next few hours. Almost without fail, they'd be on the telephone that night trying to whisper sweet nothings to get back in the good graces of their partner.

If you've ever had to deal with the tense feeling of a relationship that is going through a rough patch, you know it's hard to think of much else. How is someone supposed to succeed in recovery—a giant, new, life-altering uphill challenge—if they don't have the support, or at least don't have negativity, coming from their domestic situation?

Why do you want to leave? Because he betrayed you? Is that enough to go? For some people it is, but simply by the fact that you're reading this question in a book on this subject says to me that there is some hesitation in what you should do next.

Hesitation is good. It means that you want to gather more data before making your final decision. I'm the first to say that if you ask him to fix things, seek help, etc. and he rudely refuses and will never change, you should probably go. However, if he's trying (perhaps failing, but at least trying) to change, I hope you give him some time to prove himself.

I never had to have a "Come to Jesus" conversation with my wife, and she never laid down any new laws for the house.

Perhaps she considers herself lucky that she didn't need to do that. I fell right into line and went to work on recovery without her prompting. Your guy may not do that, but give him a little time. You may be pleasantly surprised what happens.

Is it possible to see him as anything other than a porn-obsessed monster ever again?

Tony, the mental health professional:

Yes, it is. If you're seeing him as a monster, disclosure was probably a difficult thing, perhaps even him getting caught red-handed. The last thing that I want to tell anybody in this state of mind is how they are supposed to feel right now. You probably feel that your reaction to the disclosure and your partner will never change.

Have your authentic reaction and then understand that betrayal trauma recovery is going to play a big role in your life moving forward. There's no button to push to move you past all of what's about to come with both of you putting in hard work to mend the relationship. As he begins to do his work, hopefully you will start to see more of that person you fell in love with, were drawn to, and wanted to spend the rest of your life with.

I've seen many men who legitimately have a noticeable change early in recovery. It is like the weight of the pornography addiction comes off his chest and he begins to reconnect to who he was. When this happens, women have told me they see a much-improved person, and that will help you see him as more than a "porn-obsessed monster."

Try to remember that porn addiction is not a black mark on his character, it's an illness he's probably been dealing with long before he met you. During the initial disclosure and early parts of the recovery process, it may feel natural to throw a ton of guilt and shame his way.

It's hard for me to say anything toward the betrayed in how she should initially talk to him, because she's just now learning about his addiction and trying to catch-up. I can say, "Try to be nice," but in my experience a lot of what comes out of her mouth is not pretty. Right now, I don't want her to feel like she has to filter the things she says, but I often ask women, "What is your intent with the question that you're asking? Is it legitimately to understand what led him to where he is with his addiction? Or is it for him to feel the pain that you are going through?"

I truly do understand wanting your partner to hurt the way that you have, to feel even a portion of the feelings that you are feeling, and again, I have such a difficult time telling the betrayed what they are supposed to feel, do or say. But I will say that, ultimately, what do you "win" or "gain" by wanting your partner to hurt? Unfortunately, you don't "win" a better relationship. He feels bad, and there's not truly a way to measure when or if he gets to a mark where he feels as bad as you do, so I often suggest to the couples I work with not to try and find that mark of pain equilibrium.

Josh, the former pornography addict:

That's a strong way to view him now. If you're viewing him as a monster, the initial disclosure and immediately aftermath probably didn't go well. Even if he's in complete denial and using all of the classic excuses of a porn addict, try to remember that he's a sick man.

I would work on trying to not see him as a porn-obsessed monster right now, forget the future. Whether he's your husband or boyfriend, there is something about him that you were once very fond of and fell for. If you've got this much rage, I think the first thing you have to ask yourself is if you're really mad at the man or the act of betrayal. It's a subtle difference, but it's there.

In my hometown, it was front-page news when I was arrested. As I write this, more than five years later, Amazon recently had to remove a review of my first book. I'm fine if you don't like the book, but this was a personal attack by somebody who had clearly known me prior to my arrest and has shunned me since.

While shunning is a little too Salem Witch Trials meets *The Scarlett Letter* for me, this review reflected what I've recognized for a while. There are going to be wide swaths of my community who will never see me as anything other than a porn-obsessed monster.

Everything I did leading up to my arrest, whether it be calling attention to worthwhile causes or raising thousands for them, has been erased in the eyes of those people. As it turns out, that person wasn't real, in their revised opinion, so his good deeds weren't real.

Instead, I was a liar who was hiding a secret. I don't even think their bile is about the specific crime. I think that most of them lived very sheltered, quiet, content lives, and I shook them. The guy who fought for more money in the school budget as a city councilor was also one of those cretins who looked at porn and got caught talking to a teenager. I'm long over explaining my situation, because to them, it doesn't matter. They are upset that they had to revise their truth about me.

One of the things that keeps me talking about this stuff, however, is the feedback I get from people who didn't know the old me. They don't feel like victims. They were not passively lied to for years. They just know me now as somebody trying to turn this experience into something positive.

You can either be the person who holds onto the deception, the lies, and is resentful of the new truth you must adapt to, or you can support him, even if he's still in a place of denial. I'm not saying he doesn't deserve some of your scorn, and you should obviously have your internal lie detector on when he's communicating, but he's not a monster.

He's a sick man who needs support. I'm not saying he's going to become a poster boy for porn addiction recovery or try to become the porn addiction expert I've fashioned myself as, but he can move away from this with your help.

If you're not prepared to offer help, if you're only going to see him as a monster, maybe you need some betrayal trauma recovery counseling and perspective on the entire situation. If that's impossible—and it's okay if it is—moving on may be the healthiest choice for both of you.

If I stay with him, does it mean I'm in an abusive relationship?

Tony, the mental health professional:

I've had women in sessions tell me that they always told themselves that if they caught their husband or boyfriend having a physical affair, there would be no question that they were going to leave, but with pornography, it's more complicated.

I've also had others say that they've known people who have been in a situation similar to theirs and they put up with it and didn't leave their partner. They always figured if they were in a similar situation that they would be able to put up with rebuilding things, but now that they are in the situation themselves, it feels a lot different, and some have used the word "abusive."

If he's being physically abusive that's obvious. If that's the case, you need a safety plan. Find someone who you can open up to. There is absolutely no room for physical abuse.

Admittedly, I wish society had a similar reaction for emotional abuse, but I understand that emotional abuse can be confusing, because a partner can sometimes be nice, sweet, and kind. They can say that they're never going to betray you again, or never going to yell at you again, this is the last time, this is the wake-up call that they needed to change! Have you heard that before, only to find yourself at the end of yet another verbal attack, or another conversation where you brought up something that concerned you only to have the conversation turned back on you to the point where you were apologizing, or where you were left feeling confused, or crazy? If so, please see the information on "gaslighting" that I shared at the beginning of this book. There is no place for emotional abuse, or gaslighting, in a healthy relationship either.

There are times where his addiction, or his own insecurities, may feel like a form of gaslighting or emotional abuse. I believe these are times when you may see him beat himself up emotionally, "You're right. You don't even deserve somebody like me. You might as well leave me!" This may feel like emotional abuse because it can be unproductive and can cause conversations to come to a screeching halt—or you may find yourself coming to his rescue. I believe, typically, these are signs of his own insecurities, or his own inability to confront his weakness or his addiction. In these situations, it is completely fine, even empowering, for you to set a new boundary with communication.

It is no longer acceptable for him to "run away" from the conversation by using self-deprecating statements. You may require the help of a professional to have someone keep him in the conversation without him withdrawing in order to not have to continue the discussion, "own his behaviors," or take accountability for his actions.

Take, for instance, a guy who has been conditioned to lie about his porn addiction. Now that he's been outed, it's a matter of how much do you really want or need to know? I have seen many men dig the hole they are in deeper by lying about the extent of their addiction. Why do they lie? Because they want to protect the woman, yet their actions are doing the exact same thing, causing the problem to grow, causing the gap in trust to widen.

There's no doubt that behavior is wrong, needs to be deprogrammed and causes a bigger mental scar than what was already there, but he wasn't trying to be abusive.

Finally, I would also add that if he starts to become increasingly standoffish or secretive about his recovery work, and says things like, "It's none of your business," or, "You need to get over this," it's fair to say that's a kind of emotional abuse, since he's not doing the recovery work. If he's telling you to back off despite boundaries you've set, I feel like there's some emotional abuse there. But again, simply continuing the relationship does not rise to the level of abuse in my opinion.

Josh, the former pornography addict:

You're the one who determines if you're in an abusive relationship and if you're going to stay with him. We all know blatant abuse when we see it, but if you've been in a situation that has been mainly gaslighting, I think that there certainly has been mental and emotional abuse on his part.

You're going to have friends who claim they'd leave in a second, who would never go. You'll have friends tell you to, "Stand by your man," who would be out the door in a second. You can't worry about what the others think. They're just grateful it's your dirty laundry being aired and not theirs.

Obviously, if he is getting physically abusive with you, that's something that needs to stop immediately. Stick and stones may break your bones, but fists can kill, regardless of what children's rhymes would have you believe. I'm not a supporter of staying if he's a mentally cruel man, but if he's a physically cruel man, you need to be done with this relationship ASAP.

If you find that the relationship is verbally/mentally/emotionally abusive, what steps would need to be taken to not make it abusive? Not lying to you is a good start. Sharing his feelings about his addiction, even when they may make you mad, is another.

It's important that he understand what he's doing is abuse. That message is one that can easily get lost, and if he doesn't know that his behavior rises to the level of abuse, somebody has to tell him. A professional facilitating a conversation with both of you may be the best place for that to happen.

He's either abusive or not, and that has nothing to do with if you stay with him. It has to do with his behavior and how much of it you're willing to tolerate.

Finding out he's addicted to porn has turned me off to sex completely. What should I do?

Tony, the mental health professional:

This probably goes right to the core concern that most women in this situation have, which is to wonder what they did to cause the addiction. As I've mentioned elsewhere, the answer is nothing, but that doesn't mean that there aren't going to be repercussions to not only your sex life, but also your sexual desire. It is perfectly normal for your libido to take a hit after a disclosure or discovery of porn addiction.

It's easy to believe that he lacked satisfaction in your physical appearance or in your sex life and this is why he has turned to pornography. That can cause emotional trauma involving intimacy. This is where I try to offer hope that, yes, while your intimate feelings have taken a hit, this is an opportunity to start the recovery process. If you're both willing to do the work, this is where you're going to start to build an entirely different relationship around intimacy.

Like so many other aspects of this, time is your friend, if you can be patient. It will take some time to talk through your emotions with your partner and with a professional. The more you can express your thoughts, the more you'll be able to heal.

There is some fascinating data on this subject by Dr. Kevin Skinner, one of the founders of ADDO Recovery Center in Lindon, Utah. Dr. Skinner is an expert in not only the field of pornography addiction, but also in betrayal trauma. Dr. Skinner's work shows that when we enter relationships, we're initially brought together based on the physical attraction we feel toward someone. Once we continue dating, or getting to know a new love interest, we start dealing with our deeper levels of psychological intimacy, which are honesty, trust, loyalty and commitment.

I view it almost as an "intimacy ladder." At the bottom rung is verbal intimacy. This means that, in a perfect world, we would first get to know our partner in a way in which we feel like we can talk about anything with them. We can't wait to talk to them the next day and the next. Our conversations go on for hours. We want to know everything we can about our partner, and the feeling is mutual. It's reciprocal. They, too, want to know everything they can about you!

Once you feel like the verbal intimacy is in place, you move up the ladder to emotional intimacy, meaning you can share your emotions with your partner and know that they will treat them with respect. When I'm speaking on the subject, I often say that saying your emotions with someone is like handing them your heart. What are they going to do with it? Are they going to be careful with it, delicate with it? Or are they going to throw it on the ground, stomp on it and leave it there in the street? If the former, if they're going to treat it with respect, then we now have verbal AND emotional intimacy with that partner, and we not only want to talk with them, we want to share everything with them. Next up on the ladder is cognitive and intellectual intimacy. These all play into the feelings that you're on the same page with your partner, even if one of you is a brain surgeon and another is a janitor, you still feel connected, because you have that verbal and emotional intimacy as a base. Up from there comes spiritual intimacy, which, again, if you're connected verbally, emotionally, cognitively and intellectually, then you can be in different places spiritually, but you still feel connected.

What is the top rung of the ladder, you may be asking? Physical intimacy, in my opinion, and in Dr. Skinner's work, when you are connected on all of these lower "rungs" or lower levels, then physical intimacy becomes the byproduct of being so connected. This is an entirely new, wonderful version of physical intimacy.

Too often, men with pornography addictions believe strongly that their relationship begins with a foundation of physical intimacy, and once physical intimacy is established, THEN they are willing to explore verbal, emotional, cognitive and intellectual intimacy. I maintain that the entire paradigm needs to be shifted, and there can be a lot of pushback, especially from men who have struggled with pornography and compulsive sexual behavior. They don't want to give up the, "if we just had more sex everything would be better," story that their brains are telling them. Because the truth is, more sex will not fix the marriage, it will only continue to be a "go-to" whenever they are feeling bored, lonely, angry, scared, tired, you name it. They need to change their relationship with intimacy.

I feel like it's important to note that when I work with couples, we talk about the fact that physical intimacy is absolutely a part of a healthy relationship, but increased sexual activity doesn't fix emotional scars. I'll make a bold statement. I believe that in most every marriage, a couple's entire intimacy paradigm needs to be shifted. I've had dozens and dozens of couples come in for things entirely unrelated to their intimate lives, but once we start talking, the subject of physical intimacy eventually comes up. Even in situations where people initially state that they are happy with their sex lives, upon further discovery, the relationship typically settles into a "pursuer" and a "withdrawer," or, in many cases, the wife has, over time, learned that a way to keep the peace is to give her husband sex on a regular basis, whether or not her emotional needs are being address. A healthier relationship with intimacy discussed early on in a marriage would go a long way toward improving a couple's secure connection in general.

Josh, the former pornography addict:

First, relax. I couldn't imagine a situation where this didn't have a negative effect on your sexual life. If you're like most serious couples, intercourse comes with a level of intimacy that you would never show others, and I'm not talking about making the kind of home videos that celebrities love to leak.

When you're truly in love with somebody, having sex transcends into the ultra-cheesy label of "lovemaking." Despite the fact the term is corny, the feelings are true. Now you have a partner who you have shared the most intimate, personal experiences with who has cheapened it (in your eyes) with his porn addiction.

How could you not feel a sense of betrayal? Even if he wasn't an actual sex addict, he was engaging with materials that depicted what you found so intimate and special. It's as if he's telling you that what you felt was not what he felt.

After I was found out, I think that it was actually me that had a gut-punch to the libido. My wife was able to recognize that, while the pornography was certainly a surrogate for sexual interaction, there were a lot of other things going on in my head.

I've met men and women who get hypersexual after something like this happens. I've met women who think that they need to reenact scenes from pornography in the bedroom to get the man interested, and I know of many who didn't want to touch their partner with a proverbial 10-foot pole.

I think this is an opportunity for discussion. If he's a typical addict, he probably hasn't been fully communicative with his needs or desires. I was honest with my wife that I had always been scared to death to ever request anything exotic or tell her what I liked vs. what I didn't like. I just couldn't talk about intercourse with the one person who I should be able to talk to about anything. That's on me, not her.

You need to work on your relationship and attempt to heal the betrayal that has occurred. Odds are you didn't fall in love with the guy because you thought he didn't watch pornography. I don't think being porn-free is a quality most women look for in the beginning of a relationship, although you may be regretting it now.

So why did you fall in love with him? Have those characteristics changed over time? If the answer is yes, was it because of the pornography? If they haven't changed, can you try to focus on them for a while?

You may be running through the idea in your head, "What else has he lied about?" It may be hard to feel intimate with someone who you're expecting to spring more surprises on you. It's understandable.

If you can't feel those feelings returning, speak to a professional, either with or without him. A sex-free relationship is not healthy. In rehab, I met a few women who were known as "sexual anorexics" with their anti-sex behavior. They were just as unhealthy as the full-on sex addicts. Your sex life is a spectrum, and you want to be somewhere in the middle where the healthy reside.

Chapter 8
Talking About the Addiction with Him and a Few Final Questions

How do I approach him about my suspicions?

Tony, the mental health professional:

First, know that there isn't going to be any perfect time, place, or situation that will guarantee that he will respond well to your suspicions. I have worked with a number of women who tell me that they are confident that their husband isn't being truthful about his pornography use or his inappropriate communication with other women, but they have continually put off talking about it due to upcoming family events, birthday parties, vacations, celebrations with friends, projects at work...they typically tell me that they don't want to "rock the boat" or "make things worse."

I often tell my clients that the longer they put off giving a voice to their suspicions, the longer they are delaying potential help for both them and their spouse. The longer they live with that suspicion and don't give it a chance to be discussed, the more of a wedge they may be driving between their husband and them. But this is definitely another one of those times where I completely understand the fear. I have worked with clients who have literally waited years to approach their husbands, sometimes because, as long as their suspicions aren't confirmed, they can hope that they are wrong.

It is also important to realize that there are a few different reactions that you may encounter. The best-case scenario is one where your husband immediately softens, perhaps even becomes emotional, and you can almost watch the relief wash over him as he no longer has to pretend that he can overcome this problem on his own.

More often, however, I hear of situations where the spouse will deny, deny, deny! Please understand that this is part of the behavior that has kept him from dealing with this problem more aggressively in his past. He's probably told himself that he really could stop anytime he needed to, and when confronted, his brain immediately goes into "fight or flight mode." He's choosing to fight. If he can convince you right now, in this moment, that you're wrong, then he can try once again to stop on his own.

What I fear may happen in this scenario is that he'll not only react with anger, but he may even try to convince you that you're not only wrong, but you're crazy. How dare you accuse him of something like this? Sometimes the spouse, when still in fight or flight mode, will say hurtful things, such as even if he was acting out sexually, viewing pornography or indulging in compulsive sexual behavior it was because of something that you were doing. He may say that if you were more sexually adventurous, or desired him more, then he wouldn't be doing these things in the first place. THIS IS NOT TRUE! Please do not believe that this is all your fault.

In a healthy relationship, couples should be able to bring questions, concerns, fears, and worries to their partner and have productive conversations around difficult topics. Relationships where a partner is left feeling crazy, or like they never should have brought up a topic, are not healthy, and the partner who doesn't feel like they can communicate their concerns or frustrations should seek help immediately from a professional, a religious or community leader, a parent, a sibling, or anyone they feel they can turn to and communicate with without having communication shut down.

Josh, the former pornography addict:

Carefully.

First, have a safety plan. You know this guy, or at least you think you do, but what if this is the one thing that makes him go off and get violent? Are children part of this equation?

You need to know that you can leave and stay with somebody else if he really loses it and that you have enough financial backing to allow you to be away from him while he calms down.

Yes, that's the worst case scenario, but plan for the worst and hope for the best.

My wife knew that I occasionally looked at porn, but had no idea how bad it really was. She didn't confront me because the police beat her to it, and as our lives were rapidly devolving, she wasn't all that interested in learning the ins and outs of my addictive behavior. We were too busy dodging TV cameras.

Had she decided to confront me, I would have wanted it to be as non-judgmental as possible. I would have also wanted it to be as quick as possible. Despite the fact that a high double-digits percentage of people look at pornography, nobody wants to admit it. You'd think it's a multi-billion dollar industry with no customers.

I would also want her to lay all of her cards on the table so this wouldn't be conversation one of many. I know we'd need to talk more about it in the future, but if she had already figured out her boundaries and was ready to give me certain ultimatums, I would want to hear them in the first conversation.

Don't get into the specifics of the porn. You don't really need to know why he prefers a specific type of pornography. Again, keep it as non-judgmental as possible. Whatever he's into (as long as it's legal) is his own choice and berating him for it will only turn this conversation into an argument.

Along with being non-judgmental, don't put yourself on the moral high ground. Nobody likes to be looked down upon, and nobody wants to be told, "I'm better than you." He knows his porn addiction isn't a desirable thing, and he probably wishes he could wave a magic wand and be done with it.

I know that part of the reason I hid my porn addiction from wife was so she wouldn't be hurt by it. I worried she would have been one of the women to blame herself, when the fact was I had been an addict 10 years before I met her. My faulty thinking told me that hiding the addiction was protecting her.

I would have wanted her to simply say that she was concerned about the amount of pornography I was looking at and how it was not only affecting my life, but the life of our family in general. I would have wanted her to say that she would not tolerate it in her home any longer and if she caught me again, she would tell me that I need to go stay with my parents for a while. I would have wanted to know that if I needed help dealing with my use of pornography, she would assist me in finding it, but also that it was something that needed to disappear from our lives.

That's a straightforward statement of fact that would take about 30 seconds to deliver. Notice the word "addict" is never used. She doesn't tell me how to go get help, and she clearly states what she needs and what the consequence of not meeting that need will be. There is no gray area, but also no outward judgment. I also like the fact that she put me in the driver's seat of taking care of things, but also told me she'd be there to help.

That would have been much better than incorrect newspaper stories telling the public about my addiction.

He says he's not addicted, but I think he is. What do I do?

Tony, the mental health professional:

I am a huge fan of over-communication rather than under-communication. If the wife is concerned about her husband's pornography habit, or anything that causes her to feel less connected to him, then he should welcome an opportunity to not only communicate and clear the air, but to possibly improve the relationship as he can address whatever it is that she feels is in the way.

My fear is that the couple will have two different thoughts, or feelings, about what the term addiction means. During this time, it is imperative to be able to communicate effectively, so this is probably a good conversation to have with your spouse in front of a trained professional. The key is being able to discuss the problem, your pain, your fears, your worries, and even your expectations moving forward. But that can be so difficult when emotions are high.

I once worked with a couple where the wife said that she was worried about her husband's casual attention toward their teenage daughter and her friends. Rather than expressing his shock or outrage, as I have seen in similar situations, she was able to bring it to him during a counseling session. He was visibly sad that she worried his behaviors were inappropriate, so he asked her to tell him more about what she thought she was feeling.

The husband was a hugger, and he hugged a lot of his daughter's friends. The wife opened up that she had been sexually molested by an adult who remained in her area, and she saw that adult throughout her high school years. During those times he would hug teenage girls and make them feel uncomfortable. She had never told anyone about the molestation because she worried that nobody would believe her. The husband took her hand, apologized profusely and told her he wished she had told him sooner about the molestation.

He went on to say that he had grown up without a father figure in the picture, which she was aware of. What he hadn't shared was that he had immediately stepped into the role of the "man of the house" to his four younger sisters. Growing up he wasn't always sure what to do in situations where his mother was out of the house, so he often just gave his sisters hugs and told them it would be okay. He truly felt like giving hugs was innocent.

He told her how grateful he was for her opening up to him, and he promised her that his love for her was more important than hugging girls as a greeting. He told her he had never thought of any of the girls thinking that what he was doing wasn't genuine.

In healthy relationships, couples can talk about what is bothering them and know that their partner will hear them out and try to understand where they are coming from. Your partner should want to hear what you have to say.

Josh, the former pornography addict:

Sometimes, all you can do is plant a seed, stand back and hope it germinates. If you're not the kind of person who is willing to make grand ultimatums and bring the level of confrontation up, letting him know you think he has a problem and then backing off may be the way that this has to begin. For most people, it's not a one-and-done conversation.

If he thinks he's not addicted, that's fine. It's not like there's a blood test or urine test you can force him to take that will reveal it. You may have to talk to him in a different way and not use classic terms like "addiction" when it comes to his use.

I think there are two ways to go with this:

First, you can agree with him if it's going to help the situation get resolved. Saying something like, "I respect the fact you don't think you have an addiction and you would probably know better than me, but I don't want pornography in this house and I don't want my husband looking at pornography. I feel like it disrespects me. If you continue to look at pornography, it will be hurting me and our marriage. I won't stand around and let that happen. If you don't think you can do that, either because you don't want to or you're unable, there are a lot of places that will help, but that's your decision."

Second, go the scholarly route. This is more for the person who thinks they are smart and needs facts about porn. Figure out why you think he has an addiction beyond, "He looks at a lot of porn." What negative effects has his pornography had on his life or your life together? Take a look at the definition of addiction. It may feel like you're building a PowerPoint presentation for work, but if he's anything like me, he'll accept he has an addiction once presented with the science and data.

It took me about eight days of listening to hard data regarding alcoholism at a rehab before I accepted that I had a problem with drinking. It was another six months and hundreds of hours of therapy before I was able to wrap my arms around the idea I was a pornography addict, and it was another six months before I finally accepted that addiction is a disease.

You're not going to be able to force your partner into rehab or know that he'll walk through the front door of a 12-step meeting just because you tell him it's best. Even if he accepts the fact he is an addict, the moment the words come out of his mouth, there's a lot more work that needs to be done.

You plant the seeds, you water them, you hope for sun.

He doesn't understand it hurts me. How do I make him see what he's doing is wrong?

Tony, the mental health professional:

It's unfortunate, but he's not going to completely understand what this is like for you from a betrayal trauma standpoint. Most likely he has been trying to hide this from you because of his shame, but also because he didn't want to hurt you.

No matter how softly he's confronted or how voluntarily he comes clean with his pornography addiction, you can't expect him to know what this is like for you, especially in the very beginning. He's dealing with his own complex set of shifting emotions. One of the biggest problems that I see after the initial disclosure, even if he was caught and didn't approach you voluntarily, is that once caught, he may actually begin to feel a sense of relief. This burden that he has been carrying for so long, this problem that he has been trying to overcome for sometimes years, through dozens and dozens of "this is the last time I'll do this" scenarios, is finally out in the open.

Often, he'll continue to talk about the relief he feels, and meanwhile you're trying to make sense of how he could have done this for so long without your even knowing? With each additional confession, you're going through another traumatic experience.

This is why I urge you to seek help from someone who is trained in working with betrayal trauma. An expert can help you dig deeper and hopefully help him learn to empathize with, or at least try and understand, what you're going through and what your triggers may be. An expert in betrayal trauma and/or sexual addiction, or compulsive sexual behavior, will also typically have additional assessment tools and resources to help measure the severity of the problem, which will play into the type of treatment that he, and you, may require.

There are even specific tools for disclosing the details of a sexual addiction (or affairs, both physical and emotional), all in hopes of minimizing the extent of reliving the trauma with each additional disclosure.

One of the things that I work on with couples who are dealing with the female partner's betrayal trauma recovery because of either sex or pornography addiction is to use what is called an "attachment injury apology." This term is borrowed from Sue Johnson's revolutionary couples therapy technique called "Emotionally Focused Couples Therapy" (EFT).

Attachment injury apologies arise when a spouse is triggered by an event that reminds her of the betrayal. Immediately after disclosure, these triggers can become all-encompassing, every song, smell, every place and thing, has the potential to trigger the betrayal she is now attempting to process.

Attachment injury apologies help give a voice to her triggers, and instead of just having the husband give a blanket apology, or a less-than-heartfelt apology, we work to go deeper so she knows he has some real empathy behind the apology. The apology needs to be more than "I'm sorry." He needs to try his best to understand that these triggers are now everywhere and asking her to keep them inside is exactly the wrong thing to do. She's trying to not only make sense of what she is now hearing, but also continue on the path of attempting to put a framework into place to begin to re-earn trust.

An example of this might be if the female mentions that there is a cashier at the supermarket who looks like the woman in some of the pornography she discovered on her partner's computer or telephone. Often I'll hear from a wife that she found images of women who are large breasted, particularly if she is not, or women who, as one woman said in my office, "are covered in tattoos," when she had never had a tattoo in her life. Now, the wife can be by herself, having a good day and see a large chested woman, or a woman with an arm full of tattoos, and she will immediately be triggered. Her heart rate begins to rise, her adrenaline starts flowing, her stress hormones spike, and she's livid. He's nowhere to be found, and she could be having a nervous breakdown.

When she gets home, the goal would be for her to express her triggers. If she holds them in, then she's going to continue to be angry with him, and he won't know why. She would share her experience at the store and explain that seeing a woman with large breasts or tattoos causes her to be irate.

He would say, "I am sorry that you are triggered when you see this woman at the supermarket because she reminds you of my addiction. I know this is something you have to deal with every time you go to the store, and I'm sorry that I have now put you in the position where triggers like this surround your life. I'm sorry for the pain that I've caused you that I'm aware of, and I'm especially sorry for the pain that I've caused that I'm not aware of, that you're not even yet aware of! I can't even imagine how difficult this is for you, and I'm so grateful that you're sharing this with me, even the difficult things, because I don't want you to hold things like this in."

It's important that you communicate how his behavior has negatively impacted your relationship and has caused your self-esteem to take a hit. It's fair to let him know that this has rocked the foundation of your relationship, and this might be a good time for me to remind you that ultimately the goal is healing, whether you remain together or not. I tell my clients that the wife's job moving forward is to become a trigger release valve, and his job is to become an attachment injury specialist. It's the quickest way toward healing.

I highly recommend learning this skill first inside of a therapist's office. The emotions that will initially be flowing will be intense, and you will most likely need a guide to help you through this difficult, but important process.

Josh, the former pornography addict:

Let's say for a minute that this isn't pornography. Are there other places in your life where you have put your foot down about his behavior? Maybe he was going out with his friends too often or he wasn't paying enough attention to the kids. Maybe he let the yardwork suffer or he was always late getting places. How have you resolved things in the past?

Obviously, if you can take this to couple's therapy, you'll have someone like Tony who can facilitate this better than if you handled it on your own, but if your partner isn't somebody who you can get into a room with a professional, you'll need to handle this on your own.

Is there any habit (or addiction) that you have where you might be able to put yourself into his shoes? Maybe you have issues with food, or smoking, or something that you know isn't a good thing, but you still partake. How would you want to be approached?

Once you figure out how you'd want to be approached, would anything about that approach actually prompt a change in your behavior? Would your boyfriend or husband telling you that he thinks you eat too much fried food actually stop you?

At this point, you're probably thinking, "But this is different..." Sure, it is, except it's not.

Much like I answered in the last question, I think you have to say your piece and hope that it causes change. If it doesn't, you'll have to decide what kind of ultimatums to provide and what the repercussions of not following those ultimatums will be.

The one thing I would caution you about is, depending on what phase his addiction is in, your words may mean nothing. Consider the alcoholic who reaches the point that they need to continue to drink or they could have massive health problems.

I was at the point where nobody's words would have meant anything to me once I reached the critical phase of addiction. I would have sat quietly through an intervention from my family, told them exactly what they wanted to hear, all the while knowing I was going to keep drinking and looking at pornography, not because I wanted to, but because I had to if I was going to function at all.

If he's at this point, have some compassion, even if he doesn't realize he's hurting you. If he's refusing treatment, I'd still suggest you get some counseling with a professional to plot out what your next moves are.

How do I get him to talk to me about his addiction?

Tony, the mental health professional:

I would first check your goals for having him talk about his addiction. In a perfect world, after he discloses his addiction and you both seek appropriate help, you learn new communication skills. This can be an incredible bonding experience, being able to talk about the genesis of his addiction and exploring a lot of what he has probably learned from his individual counseling. When he first viewed pornography, what was the message that he was getting from his parents, or church leaders around sexuality? Did he ever have "the talk" with his parents? How was sex discussed in the home? Did he have relatives that he heard about who were "porn addicts," and were they discussed negatively? Had he tried to stop several times in the past only to find himself back at the habit wondering, "What is wrong with me?"

But again, these types of conversations are unfortunately more of a rarity instead of the norm, especially at first. I want to normalize something I see often in my office. A wife discovers his pornography habit, or even his acting out sexually, and she is devastated. But they have kids, she wants to make it work. He is her best friend. She dives into therapy and self-help and recognizes where they lost their connection, but he has been on his way out of the relationship emotionally for a few years. This is often the time when I hear spouses say that they just want to hear about his addiction. She can be there for him. She won't use it against him. She won't judge him. Again, I understand where this is coming from.

Unfortunately, there are a couple of things at play. One, is that oftentimes when she does hear about his addiction, it bleeds into how much he was acting out in their marriage.

There are many occasions where I see the wife with the best of intentions finally hear enough, and they do eventually use the information against him with her friends or family. That can ultimately affect co-parenting. Second, the husband has been dealing with the shame of his addiction for a long time. Part of that addiction truly is the shame, fear, and isolation that leads to continually turning back to the addiction that he has tried to put behind him. His brain has basically been "trained" to NOT talk about the specifics, or to go back and revisit details, especially to his spouse. He is ashamed of his behavior, and on many occasions that is hard enough to work through even with a therapist. The addict has often spent years thinking that if they are caught, they'll die with their secrets. Often they are convinced that if they give just enough of the truth, it will suffice.

Ultimately, I would highly recommend you seek the help of a professional, because there are several important conversations that need to be had.

Typically, when a guy is feeling the guilt and shame of disclosure, then there are things that he may say to try to put his behavior back on you, or he may not take ownership of his role and seek to diminish it. If you get this kind of a response, wouldn't it be better to have a professional who has been through this and isn't on anybody's "side" to help guide the way?

You may not have to worry about this because he may be one of those guys who is relieved and you've opened the floodgates. You may be looking at long evenings of conversation as you work on this together to overcome it. Don't plan on being one of these lucky people. Most of the time, you're going to get deflection and anger if you try to bring it up.

If you're looking for a rational conversation early on in the process, you're probably going to feel like someone in the wild, lost without a map. There may have been other times in your life you've felt that way and he's been there for you, but now you're more lost than ever because he's causing this betrayal trauma.

Don't force a conversation immediately if it doesn't come naturally. He may share some things today, and more next week, and more next month. This is known as staggered disclosure, and it can do as much harm to you as anything when it comes to trauma, especially if he's claimed to tell you everything, but more information is periodically forthcoming. When they say, "I've told you everything," but repeatedly return with more, it's hard to know how to trust him.

When this staggered disclosure happens, I've seen couples fall into a pattern where the woman is now over-analyzing every word the man says and driving herself crazy trying to catch him in a lie, even in trivial parts of the disclosure.

Usually this denigrates down into a destructive communication pattern where he feels like he's trying to do the right thing and she's incapable of believing anything out of his mouth, even when it is the truth. He then gets upset that there is seemingly no way out of this cycle. It's not a good scene and can be avoided.

Being able to talk about the addiction is obviously important, but how you handle the conversations is just as important, and a specialist is advised for helping you navigate this terrain, especially in the beginning.

Josh, the former pornography addict:

The same way you talk to him about anything. Of course, it will be tense and awkward, especially at first, but this isn't like admitting you killed somebody. You're a couple and you should be able to have conversations about difficult subjects, especially when they affect the core of your relationship and the foundation it's built upon.

My wife, thankfully, didn't want the graphic details of my porn addiction, but instead wanted to know the headlines. I was able to talk to her about my addiction in broad terms, which made it much easier for me to share.

You may want to start there. The simple question, "What does addiction feel like?" is a great jumping-off point. If there are more difficult questions, you can always show empathy to attempt to get him to open up. "I think I'd be down on myself after I had looked at pornography if I didn't really want to. That must feel horrible after the fact," is a great way for him to feel like someone is relating.

The easiest place for me to talk about my addictions are either with my therapists or with fellow addicts because they understand. They don't judge, and I know I'm not going to hear words like "failure" or "pathetic" when I share my experiences. I know I won't hear them from my wife either, but we have a pretty full life without focusing on this aspect of things too critically.

It's more important that he's talking to SOMEBODY about his addiction than it is that he's talking to YOU. If he has a therapist or 12-step group, you know he's in a situation of communication that may simply feel easier than talking to you.

You're looking for a healthy partner, but that may mean that you don't fully participate in his recovery. He may want to spare you certain details or simply isn't comfortable sharing pieces of his experience with you. Try not to take it personally. Remember the goal and know that you can't plot it out like a script.

I confronted him in the past and he said he'd change, but didn't. What now?

Tony, the mental health professional:

Welcome to the world of addiction. This is the part that I always feel bad saying to the person who has been betrayed, but right now you're going to have to do a lot of the heavy lifting and set boundaries because he's been engaged in a certain pattern of behavior for a long time.

For every time he's told you he'd stop or change, he's probably told himself 100 more times. Addicts should have T-shirts that say, "This is REALLY the last time." It's not surprising when the negative pattern of behavior continues even after the disclosure.

His promise to you is likely just his way of saying, "Yes, I hear you. You don't have to keep shaming me. I will not do this again." But if he's an addict, he's going to return back to the behavior, assuming he's part of the vast majority.

This is where you have to create the boundaries. While the go-to boundary is usually leaving, it can also take the shape of not doing activities with him, separating finances, having him sleep in another room, or refusing to be intimate.

There are many times when I have heard from men who still have an unhealthy relationship with pornography that they need that release or that outlet to get through the process. It's like an alcoholic saying they just need that one drink to get through things. I don't doubt that their mind is telling them that, but you need to create a boundary. Boundaries lead to feeling more control over your emotions; boundaries can help build self-worth. Boundaries may also be the wake up that he needs to take more ownership of his actions and truly look inward to start working on the addiction from within, not by blaming others for the reason he acts out.

Regardless of what he's going through, you must make sure to take care of yourself. Set a boundary around him to make time for what you need. You're only going to make good, solid decisions if your emotional baseline is as high as possible.

Josh, the former pornography addict:

I guess I'd ask what incentive did he have to change in the past and what incentive does he have now? If you don't have boundaries, or don't follow through on your ultimatums, there is no incentive for him to listen to you give them, other than he knows it's easier to just listen and nod and then go do what he wants.

Probably about three years before the police ever got involved in my life, prior to entering the critical phase of my addiction, my wife stumbled upon my browser history after a particular session of looking at porn. She said something to the effect of, "Do you really spend this much time looking at porn?" I don't remember the exact wording, but the message I got was that I shouldn't be as involved with porn as I knew I was.

But that was the end of it. I don't know if she was asking me to change, or just making an observation, but it went in one ear and out the other because there was no incentive for me to reduce my viewing.

By the time my viewing did reach a critical point, there was nothing she could have said or done to stop me. You need to nip that in the bud before he ever gets to that place.

This sounds a little bit like a cop-out on your part. You don't think the situation can be fixed because of previous history, so why bother trying again? If you value your relationship and want it fixed, shouldn't you try again and again until you reach the conclusion it's hopeless? Once you deem it hopeless, you can either stay and brace yourself, or you can leave the relationship, but until then, you try, try, try.

If he says he'll change again, hold him to it. Find out how he's going to change. Is he going to see a therapist? Is he going to give you access to his computer? What are the ways that life will be different after you have this conversation? If he says, "You can look at my email," then look at his email.

The kind of change you're looking for needs help, and if you can be there to help him in a positive, constructive manner, you may see the change this time that you didn't before.

He says he can't stop. How am I supposed to respond to that?

Tony, the mental health professional:

With love and understanding, if at all possible. First, understand this is something he has been dealing with by himself for a long time. Just because you are now privy to his secret does not mean it can be fixed with the snap of anybody's fingers. Second, understand that he has probably promised himself, made deals with God, tried white-knuckling it, and still has been unable to stop. This may be the first time he says the words, "I can't stop," out loud, but it's not the first time he's thought them.

I've had clients say that when they get married they'll really make an effort to stop, only to find themselves returning to pornography whenever their wife is sick or in the weeks leading up to and after childbirth. Or they say that once they have a child, or get a particular job, then they'll stop. The cycle repeats itself over and over again.

Realistically, why should he believe in himself any more right now than any of the other times? You're his partner, not a miracle worker. You need to accept that, right now, he believes that the struggle will always be with him and he can't see a time where he will be able to get over his addiction.

The good news is, I've worked with enough men who have been through this to know the recovery process works. When a man commits to doing the hard work and begins to change his relationship with sex, when he starts to do things that are more fulfilling in his life (this can be career, hobbies, spending time with family) he often begins to see the connection with his wife or partner get stronger.

If he's willing to do the hard work, he can get to a place that he no longer has such a big need to check out or create the distance he once had as an active addict. But right now, it's going to feel like he can't stop and will never get his pornography addiction or compulsive sexual behaviors behind him. When you fail enough times, you can establish a pattern. But, if they do the recovery work and stay engaged with it, they can get to the point that it doesn't have the strong hold that it once did.

That being said, I have also seen guys who, because of the disclosure, suddenly feel like things are new and they can just rely on their will power this time. These are the guys who come in and say, "This time it's different," but they don't want to do the work. They may white-knuckle it and abstain for two weeks, maybe a month, but I'm typically just waiting for the relapse. This time will only be different if they put the work into it.

Men need to know that there are successes, but they are not overnight and they don't come without a lot of hard, sometimes painful, work. There may be men reading this right now who think, "Yes, that's true for others, but not me though." That's often where an addict's thinking will go. They feel that this will always be their cross to bear, and that doesn't have to be the case.

He's a Porn Addict...Now What?

Josh, the former pornography addict:

I think you need to read between the lines and figure out what he's really saying. It could be any of the following:

- I don't want to stop
- I don't think I could stop if I wanted
- I'm not going to stop
- I'm beyond hope

Now, if he's of the mindset that he's not going to stop, there's really very little you can do. The world is full of marriages that have broken up because one or both parties refuse to change. But, the good news is that refusing to change and not thinking you can change are two very different things.

I'm proof you can change, and I can introduce you to dozens of other people who are just as much proof. If he says he can't stop, what is he basing that on? Does he have some kind of unique medical condition that the rest of us didn't have?

I think what you need to do is show him it's possible. Look for success stories on the Internet that you can present to him. Urge him to attend a single meeting of Sex Addicts Anonymous just to hear from the men who have gone months and years without pornography. Introduce him to one of the many websites where men post about their struggles with pornography. Many of those sites actually have counters under the men's names to show the number of days they've abstained.

He can stop. He will have trouble, he may fall down a few times and need to pick himself up, and he may learn all kinds of things about himself along the way that he didn't know were there...and maybe that fear is also what's making him think he can't do it. He knows just how time consuming and gut-wrenching the recovery process can be. If he doesn't see his addiction as a real "problem," then why do all that work to fix it?

With alcohol, it didn't take long for me to recognize that I shouldn't just play along. I had a problem and it needed attention. It took longer than that for me to accept pornography as an issue, but once I did, I attacked it the way I attack any project: With my full attention and a strong work ethic. Recovery, when funneled in the right direction, can play to one's strengths. It can be a weird triumvirate of a job, a hobby and volunteer work. It's all in how you look at it.

If he legitimately thinks he can't do it, have him sit with a therapist for one session. If the therapist is any good, your husband or boyfriend will leave understanding that recovery is possible and that he does need it, or he will leave as stubborn as ever. Unfortunately, there are some men who would rather tear a relationship or family apart than face their demons. Your choices are to let that man live his life that way and suffer the consequences, make an effort to get him to change, or leave the situation.

Should I assume he's lying to me when he talks about his pornography use?

Tony, the mental health professional:

I'll be completely direct with you: It would be naïve not to assume he's lying because he is an addict and his addiction has been fueled by lies for years. There's a tremendous amount of guilt and shame that comes with disclosure, so I don't think there's anything wrong with having some awareness that he may not be telling you the truth. I don't think that means you have to respond around the assumption that

EVERYTHING he says is a lie, but feeling like not everything coming out of his mouth is the truth is normal.

Even if everything he is telling you is 100% true, it is normal to feel like he's lying. If it's not lying, it can be rationalization or minimizing the truth. However, voicing your belief that he's not telling you the truth might be counterproductive to your goals at this point. If you're in therapy with him, I would privately share with your therapist that you aren't trusting what he is saying and look for guidance there.

Trust issues are just one of the many reasons there is a formal disclosure process that professionals follow. One partner usually warms up to the other a little faster and feels like they can justify saying certain things or acting certain ways. That doesn't always work out as they'd hope.

If there is the staggered disclosure I mentioned in a previous question, or if he continues to be caught in lies, that's only going to retraumatize the woman, and it's important to have a therapist, perhaps even a personal one, to help navigate through these delicate waters.

Josh, the former pornography addict:

At the stage he's at, I would say 90% of what he says is going to be filtered through the lens of an addicted person. The addict knows how to manipulate, gaslight and get what they want by any means necessary.

Tony tells a story elsewhere in this book about a client who essentially lied about everything, but told the truth once. Every time he was caught in another lie, he tried to make everyone remember the time he told the truth. It's conniving, and it's classic addict behavior.

It's been explained to me this behavior is something of a survival mechanism. A person will say or do what they need to in order to get what their brain is telling them it craves. I can look back and recognize that I was also addicted to control.

I didn't necessarily need power, that was just a result of control much of the time. I wouldn't work for someone else because I needed control of the office. I needed final say of the movies that got into the film festival I co-produced because I needed control of the program. I became a journalist because I liked control of a how a story is told.

When I was at my critical worst, I wasn't talking to women in chat rooms chiefly because I got a sexual thrill. I did it because my world was crumbling around me and it was the only place I could get a sense of control.

My survival instinct told me to control a situation. Secondly, it told me to get what I needed to survive to the next day. I wasn't worried about the lies or maneuvers I was going to use on somebody next Tuesday. It was about the here and now.

I always felt it was a bonus when I could include a high percentage of truth in what I said. A benefit was that it was easier to remember things when I told the truth, and I always tried to put a kernel of truth into every lie. It's much easier to believe somebody when you can grab onto the parts of the story you know are true.

I know that you want to believe him, and trust does need to be built over time, but I'd be leery of what he says when it comes to his addiction until he has a robust plan of recovery underway.

What do I do if I think or know he looked at illegal pornography?

Tony, the mental health professional:

Thinking and knowing are two different things. If you know he's looking at illegal pornography—most likely underage—you need to alert authorities. Now that it's said, let me be frank as a therapist. I understand that people are ultimately going to have their own boundaries that they are not willing to cross. I know that some spouses are afraid to alert authorities because their entire lives will most likely be turned upside down. I can only say that if things have progressed to viewing illegal pornography, oftentimes it takes something significant to cause a change in an individual. I work with people regularly who understand, once caught, that being caught is most likely the only thing that was going to ultimately lead to their confronting the issue.

There are many women who, upon discovery of illegal pornography, will simply decide that their partner is a disgusting creep, they don't want to go any further in the relationship and they don't care what happens to their partner.

If there is any chance of you sticking around, you need to address this issue with a therapist immediately. As long as he isn't producing any of the illegal pornography, in most cases, it falls under the doctor-patient confidentiality laws. The therapist's office is a safe place if you find yourself in this position. Nobody is going to come breaking down the door.

With men who have utilized illegal pornography, they often come with a deeper, darker level of self-loathing than most addicts. If you tell them that they're a disgusting creep, it only validates what they already think about themselves.

I've heard it all behind the safety of my closed door, and when this kind of thing happens, it's important that both the female partner and I stress to the man that what he is doing is a deeper level of unhealthiness, which includes the liability of breaking the law. The potential impact that being discovered could have on the family is unthinkable and immeasurable.

The one thing I try to stress is that it can always be worse, and they are talking, which makes it easier to deal with this dark part of their addiction. This should also be discussed one-on-one between the therapist and the addict. It's important to make sure there are no signs of self-harm, including suicide.

A therapist can determine if he's any risk to himself, or others, and just how deep this part of his addiction goes.

Josh, the former pornography addict:

This is a difficult question to answer for me because it's at the heart of my case. Despite not knowing her age, I enticed a teenage girl to disrobe and perform sex acts on herself in a chat room. I was convicted for that and for taking two screenshots of her. I spent six months in jail for that.

If I had never entered those chatrooms, never gotten mixed up with something that involved a minor, where would I be today? I don't know, which makes this a difficult question to answer. I actually love where I am today. The pain is that I know I may have scarred another human being who I treated as an object for the rest of her life. I also know that my family carries a level of pain that I created. It dissipates over time for them, but it was hard on all of us. It was my fault, and it was all because I needed to see a teenager's breasts.

I found out recently that if I was seeing a therapist and I told them that I looked at underage pornography, they would not need to relate it to the police, at least not in the State of Maine. The thinking behind that is that as long as the person is not creating the pornography, there is no actual "new" victim.

I wasn't seeing a therapist at the time of my arrest, or several months earlier when I actually committed the crime. I don't think in my sickened state that I would have admitted anything about pornography to a professional at the time, but I also think that anybody who is seeing a therapist should be told what the parameters are for what can be disclosed before it is reported to officials. If a therapist is able to work with someone who can admit to looking at underage pornography and get that person to stop, isn't that better than the time, money and lives ruined to put him through the legal system?

That said, his viewing of this pornography has to stop. I think that it needs to be included as part of any speech you make about boundaries or ultimatums. He needs to know that pornography, especially that variety, will not be tolerated. I don't think it's at all out of line to tell him that if he continues looking at that variety of pornography, you will call the authorities. That may sound like a strong reaction, but if he were abusing your children, wouldn't you call the police? He doesn't get a pass because he's YOUR husband or boyfriend, or because it's not pictures of YOUR children on the screen.

There are other forms of pornography that are illegal that include torture of people or animals, and depending upon where you live, there are other genres which may violate certain decency and obscenity standards.

My wife became "that poor woman" in the question: "Why is that poor woman staying with that loser?" I have a feeling it was harder than being the loser much of the time. Do you want to be the woman in that question that people are asking every time you step into work, or the grocery store, or church?

There are lines you can cross and lines you can't cross. Your partner has crossed a line that you're not supposed to cross. You owe it to yourself, and him, to say something about this immediately and make it clear in no uncertain terms that it will not be tolerated and there will be swift action if it continues.

Do stories of porn addicts ever end with "...and they lived happily ever after?"

Tony, the mental health professional:

Absolutely they do. Unfortunately, you can't simply skip to the end of the story. There's a lot of plot development, actually character development, that needs to take place before the happily ever after, but I can honestly say that in my 15 years of working as a therapist, primarily in the world of pornography addiction and compulsive sexual behavior, MOST of the couples I see get to a point in therapy where they admit that, had there not been disclosure or had their partner not gotten caught, they never would have learned the skills that allow them to connect in an entirely different, more healthy way.

There is a lot of work ahead of you that will probably be extremely difficult, yet incredibly rewarding. As a couple's therapist, I have seen so many people end their journey with me in a better relationship that has deeper intimacy and more open communication than they've ever experienced in their relationship prior.

An important piece to highlight is that "happily ever after" is not "the way it was at the beginning of the relationship." Those may have been happy times, but everything that bubbled to the surface was already there, waiting to come out.

When I wrap things up with these couples, one of them inevitably says what the other is thinking and what I've heard so many times: "I never thought that we would ever be here as a couple, and it never would have happened had it not been through the disclosure of pornography addiction."

If you're going to end up "happily ever after," you need to develop the tools to get there and to stay there. Helping couples get to that spot is one of the most rewarding things about my job. When people arrive, they are usually two individuals barely in a relationship, but if they successfully do the work, they get to the point where they are one couple deep in a relationship.

In going through the healing process, you're going to learn a lot about yourself and a lot about your partner that you never knew was there. You'll learn how to communicate without judgment, learn how to feel and express empathy, and develop a keener awareness about your partner than you've ever had. When the couple gets to that point, and continues practicing the tools they've learned, it's pretty darn close to "happily ever after" beyond that.

Josh, the former pornography addict:

Does anybody's? At this point, I'm just hoping for, "...and they lived as contently as they could given what was thrown at them from time-to-time."

I worked briefly with a woman who was very nice, but she seemed hellbent on sticking to some script that she created in her head probably around the age of 9. It involved a perfect childhood, followed by four years of college, marrying her childhood sweetheart, finding purpose in her work, having two kids and building the house of her dreams.

I don't know what happens beyond that, but she had this script mapped out and she was not going to deviate. When slight deviations would occur, it would somehow morph into part of the original story and become what she wanted all along.

While I haven't been on social media since the day of my arrest—nor do I ever plan to go back, other than as an avenue for marketing and advertising my professional endeavors—my wife has pointed out to me on more than one occasion that this woman still likes to post comments about how perfect her "fairytale life" has come out.

I'm genuinely unsure if she thinks she's a princess or if she's in a secret hell and overcompensating with unrealistic shares. Either way, there's probably a giant fall coming at some point in her life that she's unready for.

When things were going very well for me, I don't think my wife or I tried to pretend we were the perfect couple or had the perfect life, because it would have been too much energy wasted on appearances. Neither of us had the spare time or desire to attempt creation of jealousy in others, and despite the attention I craved from the world, neither of us needed affirmation that we were living happily ever after.

So, I will say, no porn addict's life ends with, "...and they lived happily ever after," but that is because I don't think anybody's life does.

I can, however, say that along with living as contently as we can with the occasional hiccups, we're living better than we ever have, and I'd even say better than I ever thought realistically possible.

Not only can it go back to where it was, it can get better than ever before.

What Did You Think of This Book?

First of all, thank you for purchasing this book. We know you could have picked any number of books to read, but you picked this book and for that we are extremely grateful.

We hope that it added at value and quality to your everyday life. If so, it would be really nice if you could share this book with your friends and family by posting to Facebook and Twitter.

If you enjoyed this book and found some benefit in reading this, we would like to hear from you and hope that you could take some time to post a review on Amazon, Barnes & Noble, or Goodreads. Your feedback and support will help us improve the books we publish. If you would like to leave a copy of your review (or a review not posted elsewhere) on our blog, you can follow this link to leaiving your book review as a comment now.

We wish you all the best in your future success!

Select MSI Books

Inspirational and Religious Books

A Believer-in-Waiting's First Encounters with God (Mahlou)

A Guide to Bliss: Transforming Your Life through Mind Expansion (Tubali)

Christmas at the Mission: A Cat's View of Catholic Beliefs and Customs (Sula)

Easter at the Mission: A Cat's Observation of the Paschal Mystery (Sula)

El Poder de lo Transpersonal (Ustman)

Everybody's Little Book of Everyday Prayers (MacGregor)

How to Argue with an Atheist: How to Win the Argument without Losing the Person (Brink)

Introductory Lectures on Religious Philosophy (Sabzevary)

Jesus Is Still Passing By (Easterling)

Joshuanism (Tosto)

Living in Blue Sky Mind: Basic Buddhist Teachings for a Happy Life (Diedrichs)

One Family: Indivisible (Greenebaum)

Overcoming the Odds (C. Leaver)

Puertas a la Eternidad (Ustman)

Saints I know (Sula)

Surviving Cancer, Healing People: One Cat's Story (Sula)

Memoirs

57 Steps to Paradise: Finding Love in Midlife and Beyond (Lorenz)

Blest Atheist (Mahlou)

Forget the Goal, the Journey Counts . . . 71 Jobs Later (Stites)

From Deep Within: A Forensic and Clinical Psychologist's Journey (Lewis)

One Simple Text... (Shaw & Brown)

Good Blood: A Journey of Healing (Schaffer)

Healing from Incest: Intimate Conversations with My Therapist (Henderson & Emerton)

It Only Hurts When I Can't Run: One Girl's Story (Parker)

Las Historias de Mi Vida (Ustman)

Of God, Rattlesnakes, and Okra (Easterling)

Tucker and Me (Harvey)

Psychology & Philosophy

Anger Anonymous: The Big Book on Anger Addiction (Ortman)

Anxiety Anonymous: The Big Book on Anxiety Addiction (Ortman)

Awesome Couple Communication (Pickett)

Depression Anonymous: The Big Book on Depression Addiction (Ortman)

El Poder de lo Transpersonal (Ustman)

Harnessing the Power of Grief (Potter)

Road Map to Power (Husain & Husain)

The Marriage Whisperer: How to Improve Your Relationship Overnight (Pickett)

The Rose and the Sword: How to Balance Your Feminine and Masculine Energies (Bach & Hucknall)

The Seven Wisdoms of Life (Tubali)

Understanding the Analyst: Socionics in Everyday Life (Quinelle)

Understanding the Critic: Socionics in Everyday Life (Quinelle)

Understanding the Entrepreneur: Socionics in Everyday Life (Quinelle)

Understanding the People around You: An Introduction to Socionics (Filatova)

Understanding the Romantic (Quinelle)

Understanding the Seeker: Socionics in Everyday Life (Quinelle)

Self-Help Books

100 Tips and Tools for Managing Chronic Illness (Charnas)

A Woman's Guide to Self-Nurturing (Romer)

Creative Aging: A Baby Boomer's Guide to Successful Living (Vassiliadis & Romer)

Divorced! Survival Techniques for Singles over Forty (Romer)

Helping the Disabled Veteran (Romer)

How to Get Happy and Stay That Way: Practical Techniques for Putting Joy into Your Life (Romer)

How to Live from Your Heart (Hucknall) (Book of the Year Finalist)

Life after Losing a Child (Young & Romer)

Publishing for Smarties: Finding a Publisher (Ham)

Recovering from Domestic Violence, Abuse, and Stalking (Romer)

RV Oopsies (MacDonald)The Widower's Guide to a New Life (Romer)(Book of the Year Finalist)

Widow: A Survival Guide for the First Year (Romer)

Widow: How to Survive (and Thrive!) in Your 2d, 3d, and 4th Years (Romer)

CPSIA information can be obtained
at www.ICGtesting.com
Printed in the USA
LVHW052131021219
639122LV00003B/94